PRACTICAL MANAGEMENT OF HYPERTENSION

W0050458

PRACTICAL MANAGEMENT OF HYPERTENSION

edited by
Willem H. Birkenhäger

Professor of Medicine
Erasmus University, Rotterdam, The Netherlands

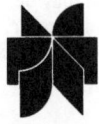

SPRINGER SCIENCE+BUSINESS MEDIA, B.V.

British Library Cataloguing in Publication Data

Practical management of hypertension.
  1. Man. Blood. Hypertension
  I. Birkenhäger, W. H. (Willem H.)
  616.132

Library of Congress Cataloging in Publication Data

Practical management of hypertension / edited by Willem H. Birkenhäger.
     p. cm.
  Includes bibliographical references.
  Includes index.
  ISBN 978-94-010-5655-7   ISBN 978-94-011-3724-9 (eBook)
  DOI 10.1007/978-94-011-3724-9
  1. Hypertension. I. Birkenhäger, W. H.
  [DNLM: 1. Cardiovascular Diseases. 2. Hypertension. 3. Hypertension--therapy.
  4. Risk Factors. WG 340 P8955]
  RC685.H8P73 1990
  616.1'32--dc20
  DNLM/DLC
  For Library of Congress   90-5352
                                                   CIP

Contents

CONTENTS

List of first authors

Dr Gaston E. Bauer
Department of Cardiology
Royal North Shore Hospital
ST LEONARDS NSW 2065
Australia

Professor Lawrence J. Beilin
University of Western Australia
35 Victory Square
PERTH WA 6000
Australia

Professor Willem H. Birkenhäger
Erasmus University
ROTTERDAM
The Netherlands

Dr Frans Boomsma
Department Internal Medicine I
University Hospital Dijkzigt
Dr. Molewaterplein 40
3015 GD ROTTERDAM
The Netherlands

Professor Armin Distler
Department of Internal Medicine
Clinic Steglitz
Free University
D-1000 BERLIN 45
FRG

Professor Lennart Hansson
Department of Medicine
University of Göteborg
Hospital Östra
S-41685 GÖTEBORG
Sweden

Professor Gastone Leonetti
Center of Physiology
Hypertension Clinic
Hospital Maggiore
Via F. Storza 35
I-20122 MILAN
Italy

Dr Eoin O'Brien
The Blood Pressure Unit
Beaumont Hospital
DUBLIN 9
Eire

Dr Roger A. Shinton
University of Birmingham
Department of Medicine
Dudley Road Hospital
BIRMINGHAM B18 7QH
UK

Dr Jan Staessen
Clinical Laboratory Hypertension
Internal Medicine – Cardiology
University Hospital Gasthuisberg
Herestraat 49, B-3000 LEUVEN
Belgium

Introduction

WILLEM H. BIRKENHÄGER

This compact guide aims to define the current approach to hypertension in practice, with the focus on the individual whom the physician faces across his desk.

In the population, blood pressures are distributed along a Gaussian type of curve, but with some tailing towards the upper range.

A systolic blood pressure of 160 mmHg is commonly accepted as the upper limit of the normal range. For diastolic pressure, the gradings are much more detailed: borderline hypertension (90–94 mmHg, mild hypertension (95–104 mmHg), moderate hypertension (105–114 mmHg), and severe hypertension (115 mmHg and over). Despite its skewing to the right, the bell shape of the distribution curve of blood pressures implies that the milder elevations of blood pressure are the most common. Such pressures are observed in 15–20% of the population upon casual measurement. After rechecking – which is mandatory – the prevalence of hypertension drops to some 5%, due to psychological and statistical factors. Even this modest segment of the population represents an important proportion in terms of future cardiovascular risk. It is an essential part of preventive and curative health care to identify these people; the more so, because some 40% of the excess risk has already been proven to be reversible by conventional antihypertensive treatment.

The individual dividends of treatment logically tend to increase pari passu with the initial risk level, which is compounded by blood pressure stratum, age, (male) gender, positive family history of hypertensive complications, hypercholesterolaemia, smoking, etc. Although blood pressure per se obviously is just part of the risk profile, it serves as the most convenient gate to a further appraisal of the full prognostic cardiovascular profile. The family practitioner finds himself in a uniquely suitable position, in that he can afford to tread gently but persuasively, while carrying a big therapeutic stick, to paraphrase Theodore Roosevelt.

I feel deeply indebted to the authors, who have contributed to this work with a great deal of compassion and enthusiasm. They share a vast experience in exploring the interface between clinical science and practical issues. Their Chapters without exception reflect the purpose of this lean and pragmatic vademecum. Even within the sober framework of this book, some overlaps and controversies between chapters proved to be unavoidable. I have tried to minimize overlaps as much as possible by eliminating obvious redundancies and inserting cross-references instead. Controversial points of view have been left untouched in the interests of stimulating curiosity and encouraging further reading. To the latter purpose the authors were asked to limit their reference lists to brief selections of key papers instead of preparing fully referenced texts.

The authors hope that the practicing physician will recognize his working conditions and his recurrent dilemmas when he peruses these contents; it would be a gratifying thought if he would feel supported in one way or another in his management of the hypertensive individual.

Willem H. Birkenhäger, MD, PhD
Professor of Medicine
Erasmus University

Rotterdam, May 1990

CHAPTER 1

Techniques for measuring blood pressure and their interpretation

EOIN O'BRIEN and KEVIN O'MALLEY

INTRODUCTION

There are many techniques for measuring blood pressure. In clinical practice the most commonly used of these is auscultation of the Korotkov sounds during deflation of an occluding cuff attached to a mercury sphygmomanometer. In this review most attention will be directed, therefore, to this well-established but much-misused technique. Other methods, such as oscillometry, are becoming increasingly popular and these will be given briefer consideration. Developing techniques, such as plethysmography, will be mentioned but not afforded any great detail. The emphasis of the chapter will be on the clinical measurement of blood pressure and the mechanisms of blood pressure detection will not be considered.

THE CONVENTIONAL TECHNIQUE OF BLOOD PRESSURE MEASUREMENT

The measurement of blood pressure in clinical practice is dependent on the accurate transmission and interpretation of a signal (Korotkov sound or pulse wave) from a *subject* via a device (the *sphygmomanometer*) to an *observer*. The successful outcome of this complex interaction requires that the observer is competent in performing the *technique* of blood pressure measurement. The procedure is fraught with sources of potential error which may arise in the observer, the subject, the sphygmomanometer or in the overall application of the technique.

1

The observer

It is logical to open discussion with the observer, who in practice may be a doctor, nurse, health worker or even a patient. Whereas it is accepted without reservation that patients, paramedical personnel, and, perhaps to a lesser degree, nurses must receive detailed instruction in blood pressure measurement, in medical schools the student, after some theoretical instruction, is expected to 'acquire' the necessary skills for the performance of the technique. We have, therefore, two problems: *first*, to determine what constitutes adequate training and, *second*, to devise a means of assessing the efficacy of that training.

Observer error

In 1964, Geoffrey Rose and his colleagues classified observer error into three categories; systematic error, terminal digit preference and observer prejudice.

Systematic error may be caused by lack of mental concentration, deteriorating auditory acuity, confusion of auditory and visual cues, etc., but the most important factor is failure to interpret accurately the Korotkov sounds, especially for diastolic pressure.

Terminal digit preference refers to the phenomenon whereby the observer rounds off the pressure reading to a digit of his or her chosing, most often to zero.

Observer prejudice or *bias* is the practice whereby the observer simply adjusts the pressure to meet his or her preconceived notion of what the pressure should be.

Training techniques

Various methods and techniques have been used to achieve greater accuracy in blood pressure measurement. These include direct instruction, manuals and booklets, audiotapes and video films. Of these the most effective combination is direct instruction using a video film. Video films generally use the method devised by Wilcox which consists of a series of blood pressure recordings in which a mercury column is seen falling in concert with recorded Korotkov sounds. The observer is required to record the level of mercury in the column corresponding to the systolic and diastolic pressures. A number of the recordings are duplicated unknown to the trainee observer so that within-observer reliability can be tested. The reference pressure is determined from the mean scores of a number of expert observers.

Recently, the Working Party on Blood Pressure Measurement of the British Hypertension Society (BHS) has produced a film which incorporates the method just described but, in addition, the first part of the film is devoted to a visual presentation of the BHS recommendations on blood pressure measurement. Using the BHS film combined with direct instruction we have been able to bring paired nurse observer measurements within 5 mmHg of each other for both systolic and diastolic pressure.

The sphygmomanometer

The sphygmomanometer is an indispensable piece of diagnostic medical equipment. The mercury sphygmomanometer has served us well since blood pressure measurement was first introduced into clinical practice, but all too often its continuing efficiency is taken for granted. An aneroid manometer may be substituted for the mercury column but is generally not as reliable. Both devices are used to measure blood pressure by auscultation and a stethoscope is also required.

There are many semi-automated and automated devices on the market but few of these have been adequately tested for accuracy and reliability and those which have been evaluated have been shown generally to be too inaccurate for clinical practice.

The device

Mercury sphygmomanometers

The mercury sphygmomanometer is the simplest, most accurate and most economical device for the indirect measurement of blood pressure and stands, at the time of writing, as the recommended device for the clinical measurement of blood pressure. It can be maintained and serviced easily without having to be returned to the supplier but users should be alert to the hazards associated with handling mercury. The criteria opposite must be fulfilled in order to obtain the most accurate measurements with a mercury sphygmomanometer:

TIPS FOR CHECKING THE MERCURY METER

* The top of the mercury meniscus should rest at exactly zero without pressure applied; if it is below this, mercury should be added to the reservoir.

* The scale should be clearly calibrated in 2 mm divisions from 0 to 300 mmHg and should indicate accurately the differences between the levels of mercury in the tube and in the reservoir.

* The diameter of the reservoir must be at least 10 times that of the vertical tube, or the vertical scale must correct for the drop in the mercury level in the reservoir as the column rises.

* Substantial errors may occur if the manometer is not kept vertical during measurement. Calibrations on floor models are especially adjusted to compensate for the tilt in the face of the gauge. Stand-mounted manometers are recommended for hospital use. This allows the observer to adjust the level of the sphygmomanometer and to perform measurement without having to balance the sphygmomanometer precariously on the side of the bed.

* The air vent at the top of the manometer must be kept patent as clogging will cause the mercury column to respond sluggishly to pressure changes and to overestimate pressure.

* The control valve is one of the commonest sources of error in sphygmomanometers and when it becomes defective it should be replaced. Spare control valves should be available in hospitals and a spare control valve should be supplied with sphygmomanometers.

Aneroid manometers

Aneroid sphygmomanometers register pressure through a bellows and lever system which is mechanically more intricate than the mercury reservoir and column. Their accuracy is affected by the jolts and bumps of everyday use and they lose accuracy over time leading usually to false low readings and a consequent underestimation of blood pressure. They are less accurate than mercury sphygmomanometers.

Aneroid sphygmomanometers must be checked every six months against an accurate mercury sphygmomanometer over the entire pressure range. This may be done by connecting the aneroid sphygmomanometer with a Y piece to the tubing of mercury sphygmomanometer and inflating the cuff around a bottle or cylinder. If inaccuracies or other faults are found, the instrument must be returned to the manufacturer or supplier for repair.

Semi-automated and automated devices

One consequence of the increased interest in blood pressure measurement has been the creation of a large market for blood pressure measuring devices. A number of semi-automated devices based on Korotkov sound detection are available. An electronic microphone, in the pressure cuff, shielded from extraneous noise in the pressure cuff is used to detect the Korotkov sounds and blood pressure may be recorded on a chart or indicated on a digital display. The microphones are sensitive to movement and friction, however, and may be difficult to place accurately. Manual or automatic inflation and deflation, or both, may be available. In recent years the number of devices available commercially has risen rapidly but most have been shown to be inaccurate when compared with the mercury sphygmomanometer, though some have been found to be satisfactory. Most semi-automated devices work on one of three principles – the detection of Korotkov sounds by a microphone or the detection of arterial blood flow by ultrasound or oscillometry. Other techniques which have been tried or are being developed include the phase-shift method; infrasound recording; wide-band external pulse recording; plethysmography, tonometry and ultrasound, but as with other automated devices the results of validation have often been disappointing. At present there is no obligation on manufacturers to comply with the few recommended standards that are available.

The cuff and bladder

The cuff

The cuff is an inelastic cloth that encircles the arm and encloses the inflatable rubber bladder. It is secured round the arm most commonly by means of Velcro on the adjoining surfaces of the cuff, occasionally by wrapping a tapering end into the encircling cuff, and rarely by hooks. Tapering cuffs should be long enough to encircle the arm several times: the full length should extend beyond the end of the inflatable bladder for 25 cm and then should gradually taper for a further 60 cm. Velcro surfaces must be effective, and when they lose their grip the cuff should be discarded. It should be possible to remove the bladder from the cuff so that the latter can be washed from time to time.

The inflatable bladder

Of the many controversial issues in hypertension few can rival that of determining the optimal bladder dimensions for a particular arm circumference. It is fair to say that a review of the sizable literature on the subject often serves to confuse rather than clarify.

It is generally agreed that the width of the bladder is not as critical as the length provided bladder length is adequate and the bladder is not excessively narrow. For most adult arms a width of 12–14 cm is adequate. The main argument centres on bladder length. The American Heart Association recommend the so-called 'standard' cuff containing a bladder with dimensions of 12 × 23 cm for non-obese arms, and cuffs containing larger bladders for obese subjects. However, the overwhelming opinion from the literature is for bladders with greater lengths (32–42 cm) so that the arm is encircled by the bladder in most subjects.

The American Heart Association recommends that five cuffs should be available for blood pressure measurement. However justifiable these recommendations may be on theoretical grounds, the provision of such a large variety of cuff sizes is clearly not feasible in practice. Moreover, these recommendations incorporate measurement of the arm circumference as a fundamental feature of blood pressure measurement which, it may be argued, is already a complex-enough technique. The recommendations may be further faulted on the basis that most adult arms will not readily accomodate cuffs containing bladders with widths exceeding 13 cm because the cuff encroaches on the antecubital fossa and interferes with auscultation.

The British Hypertension Society and the British Standards Institution have each decided to simplify matters by recommending only three cuffs (Table I) for routine clinical use with the proviso that for very large arms care should be taken to ensure that the centre of the bladder is placed over the brachial artery. All cuffs should be imprinted with a clear white line indicating the centre of the inflatable bladder. This recommendation has taken account of the occurrence of different arm size is in the adult population and it has been calculated that a cuff containing a bladder 35 cm long would encircle 99% of adult arms.

Table 1. Recommended bladder dimensions

Dimensions (cm)	Subject	Maximum arm circumference
13 × 4	Small children	17 cm
18 × 8	Medium-sized children	26 cm
35 × 12.5	Grown children & adults	42 cm

Accurate readings may be obtained in adults with arm circumferences greater than 42 cm by placing a cuff with a 35 cm bladder so that the centre of the bladder is over the brachial artery

(Reproduced from *Blood Pressure Measurement* by permission of the *British Medical Journal*)

Inflation–deflation system

The inflation–deflation system consists of an inflating and deflating mechanism connected by rubber tubing to an occluding bladder. Automated devices, of which there are many varieties, operate on the principle that once the device has been activated, it inflates automatically to a programmed cuff pressure and then deflates, automatically sensing the blood pressure, most commonly with a microphone, but increasingly by oscillometry and ultrasound. The recorded pressure may then be stored and/or displayed on a screen or printed.

The standard mercury and aneroid sphygmomanometers used in clinical practice are operated manually with inflation being effected by means of a bulb compressed by hand and deflation by means of a release valve which is also controlled by hand. The pump and control valve are connected to the inflatable bladder and thence to the sphygmomanometer by rubber tubing.

Rubber tubing: Leaks due to cracked or perished rubber make accurate measurement of blood pressure difficult because the fall in mercury cannot be controlled. The rubber should be in a good condition and free from leaks. The minimum length of tubing between the cuff and the manometer should be 70 cm and, between the inflation source and the cuff, the tubing should be at least 30 cm in length. Connections should be airtight and easily disconnected.

Control valve: One of the most common sources of error in sphygmo-manometers is the control valve, especially when an air filter rather than a

7

rubber valve is used. When defective it may cause leakage, making it difficult to control the release of pressure, which thus leads to underestimation of systolic and overestimation of diastolic pressure. The filter in the valve may become blocked with dirt, which demands excessive squeeze on the pump. The control valve should allow the passage of air without excessive effort; when closed it should hold the mercury at a constant level, and when released it should allow a controlled fall in the level of mercury. Faults in the control valve may be corrected easily and cheaply, sometimes by simply cleaning the filter or alternatively by replacing the control valve.

Stethoscope

The stethoscope should be a high-quality one in good condition with clean, well-fitting earpieces. The bell is most suited to the auscultation of low-pitched sounds, such as the Korotkov sounds, but in routine blood pressure measurement it probably does not matter much whether the bell or diaphragm is used provided the stethoscope is placed over the palpated brachial artery in the antecubital fossa. In fact, because the diaphragm covers a greater area and is easier to hold than a bell endpiece it is reasonable to recommend it for routine clinical measurement of blood pressure.

Maintenance

Mercury sphygmomanometers are easily checked and maintained but care should be taken when handling mercury. Mercury sphygmomanometers need cleaning and checking at least every six months in hospital use and every 12 months in general practice.

Technique

Blood pressure measurement is one of the few scientific measurements undertaken by doctors in the course of clinical assessment and it occupies more of the nurse's time, on the wards, in the accident and emergency department and in the out-patients departments, than any other measurement. The situation is similar in family practice. The consequences of decisions arising from the measurement of blood pressure may be crucial to patient management in the short-term and, perhaps more importantly, the level of blood pressure recorded may influence the quality of existence for the remainder of a patient's life. It follows, therefore, that considerable care should be given to the technique of blood pressure measurement. The following guidelines to performing the technique are drawn mostly from the *ABC of Hypertension* and the *British Hypertension Society Recommendations on Blood Pressure Measurement*.

Variability of blood pressure

The observer must be aware of the considerable variability that may occur in blood pressure from moment to moment with respiration, emotion, meals, tobacco, alcohol, temperature, bladder distension and pain, and that blood pressure is also influenced by age, race and circadian variation. It is not always possible to modify these many factors but we can minimise their effect by taking them into account in reaching a decision as to the relevance or otherwise of a particular blood pressure measurement.

Insofar as is practical the patient should be relaxed in a quiet room at a comfortable temperature and a short period of rest should precede the measurement. When it is not possible to achieve optimum conditions, this should be noted with the blood pressure reading – for example, 'BP 154/92, R arm, V phase (patient very nervous)'.

The defence reaction: 'white coat hypertension'

Anxiety raises blood pressure, often by as much as 30 mmHg. The defence or alarm reaction is a rise in blood pressure associated with blood pressure measurement. This increase in blood pressure may subside once the subject becomes accustomed to the procedure and the observer, but in many subjects blood pressure is always higher when measured by doctors, and to a lesser degree by nurses – so-called 'white coat hypertension'.

Explanation to subject

The first step, therefore, in blood pressure measurement is adequate explanation of the procedure in an attempt to allay fear and anxiety, especially of nervous subjects. In particular, subjects having blood pressure measured for the first time should be told that there is minor discomfort caused by inflation of the cuff.

9

Attitude of observer

The observer should have been trained as discussed previously. Before taking the blood pressure, he or she should be in a comfortable relaxed position. If the observer is hurried the pressure will be released too rapidly with under-estimation of systolic and overestimation of diastolic pressures. If there is interruption the exact measurement may be forgotten and an approximation made. Therefore, the blood pressure should be written down as soon as it has been measured; relying on memory may result in error.

Posture of subject

Posture affects blood pressure with a general tendency for it to increase from the lying to sitting or standing position. However, in most people posture is unlikely to lead to significant error in blood pressure measurement provided the arm is supported at heart level. Nonetheless, it is advisable to standardise posture for individual patients and in practice blood pressure is usually measured in the sitting position. Patient should be comfortable whatever their position. No information is available on the optimal time that a subject should remain in a particular position before a measurement, but three minutes is suggested for the lying and sitting positions and one minute standing. Some antihypertensive drugs cause postural hypotension, and when this is expected blood pressure should be measured both lying and standing.

Arm support

If the arm in which measurement is being made is unsupported, as tends to happen if the subject is sitting or standing, isometric exercise is performed raising blood pressure and heart rate. Diastolic blood pressure may be raised by as much as 10% by having the arm extended and unsupported during blood pressure measurement. The effect of isometric exercise is greater in hypertensive patients and in those taking β-adrenoceptor blocking drugs. It is essential, therefore that the arm is supported during blood pressure measurement and this is best achieved in practice by having the observer hold the subject's arm at the elbow (Fig. 1) though in research the use of an arm support on a stand has much to commend it.

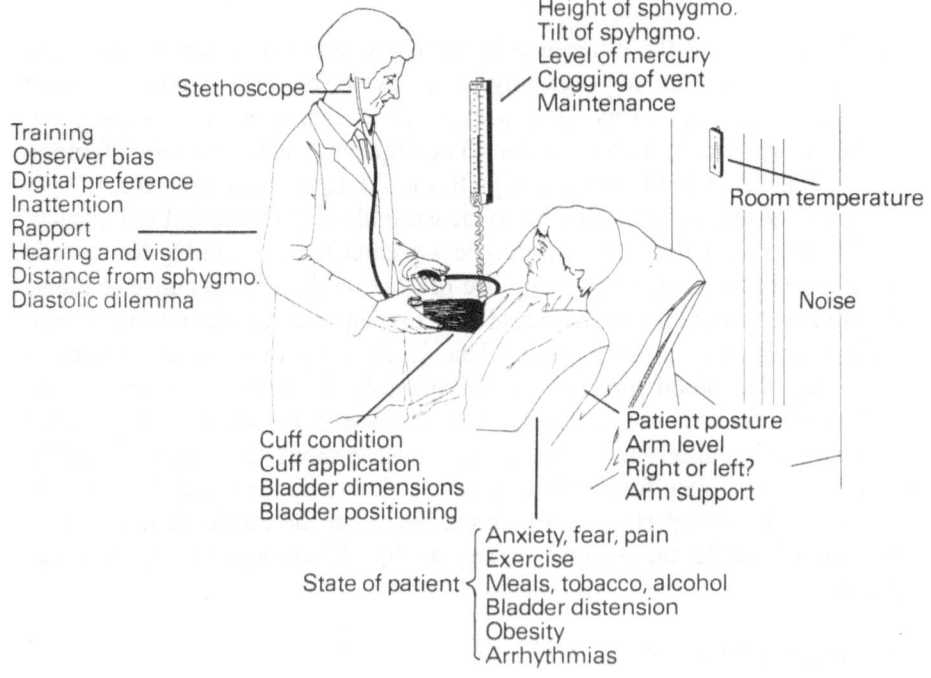

Stethoscope

Height of sphygmo.
Tilt of spyhgmo.
Level of mercury
Clogging of vent
Maintenance

Training
Observer bias
Digital preference
Inattention
Rapport
Hearing and vision
Distance from sphygmo.
Diastolic dilemma

Room temperature

Noise

Cuff condition
Cuff application
Bladder dimensions
Bladder positioning

Patient posture
Arm level
Right or left?
Arm support

State of patient ⎨ Anxiety, fear, pain
Exercise
Meals, tobacco, alcohol
Bladder distension
Obesity
Arrhythmias

Fig. 1. Overview of the arrangements for measuring blood pressure

Arm position

Not only should the arm be supported but it must also be horizontal at the level of the heart as denoted by the mid-sternal level. Dependency of the arm below heart level leads to an overestimation of systolic and diastolic pressures and raising the arm above heart level leads to underestimation of these pressures. The magnitude of this error can be as great as 10 mmHg for systolic and diastolic pressures. This source of error becomes especially important in the sitting and standing positions when the arm is likely to be dependent by the subject's side. However, it has recently been demonstrated that even in the supine position an error of 5.5 mmHg for diastolic pressure may occur if the arm is not supported at heart level.

Which arm?

The significance of the difference in blood pressure between arms has been the subject of debate for over fifty years. However, early studies showing differences between arms used sequential measurement and subsequent studies using simultaneous, rather than sequential measurement of blood pressure, have tended to show no significant difference between arms.

A reasonable policy would be to measure blood pressure in both arms at the initial examination, and if differences greater than 20 mmHg for systolic or 10 mmHg for diastolic pressure are present on three consecutive readings simultaneous measurement should be carried out to determine if the difference is real or artefactual. This is done by two trained observers recording the blood pressure simultaneously in both arms using one sphygmomanometer connected by a Y connector to two occluding cuffs. When there is a difference between arms a cause should be sought and in the absence of any being found blood pressure should be recorded thereafter in the arm with the highest pressure on the basis that the cardiovascular system may be subject to the adverse effects of the higher rather than the lower pressure.

Application of the cuff

Bulky, tight or restrictive clothing should be removed from the arm. If a blouse, shirt, or pyjama jacket is worm it is better to leave the cloth under the cuff rather than roll the sleeve into a constricting band. If the cuff is not applied snugly to the arm falsely high blood pressures will be recorded, and if the cuff is too tight errors may also occur.

The cuff should be wrapped round the arm ensuring that the bladder dimensions are accurate. If the bladder does not completely encircle the arm the centre of the bladder must be over the brachial artery. The rubber tubes from the bladder are usually placed inferiorly, often at the site of the brachial artery, but it is now recommended that they should be placed superiorly or, with completely encircling bladders, posteriorly, so that the antecubital fossa is easily accessible for auscultation. The lower edge of the cuff should be 2–3 cm above the point of brachial artery pulsation (Fig. 2).

Position of manometer

The observer should be no further than three feet from the manometer so that the scale can be read easily. The mercury manometer has a vertical scale and errors will occur unless the eye is kept close to the level of the meniscus. The aneroid scale is a composite of vertical and horizontal divisions and numbers and must be viewed straight on with the eye on a line perpendicular to the centre of the face of the guage. The mercury column should be vertical (although some models are designed with a tilt) and at eye level – this is achieved most effectively with stand-mounted models which can be easily adjusted to suit the height of the observer (Fig. 1).

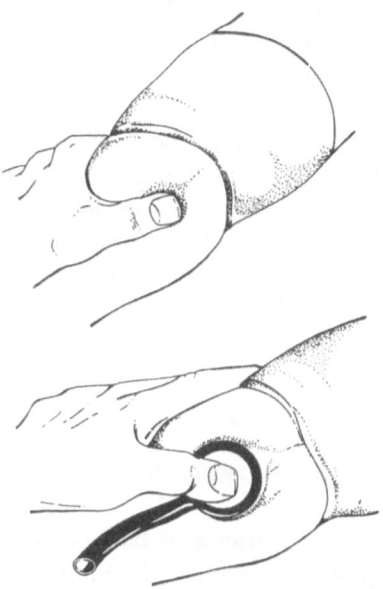

Fig. 2. Correct position of (inflated) cuff. Palpation and auscultation of brachial artery

Palpatory estimation of blood pressure

The brachial artery should be palpated while the cuff is rapidly inflated to about 30 mmHg above the disappearance of the pulse and then slowly deflated. The observer should note the pressure at which the pulse reappears. This is the approximate level of the systolic pressure, and because Phase I sounds sometimes disappear as pressure is reduced and reappear at a lower level (the auscultatory gap), the systolic pressure may be underestimated unless already determined by palpation. The palpatory technique is also useful in patients in whom auscultatory end points may be difficult to judge accurately – for example, pregnant women, patients in shock, or those taking exercise. (The radial artery is often used for palpatory estimation of the systolic pressure but by using the brachial artery the observer also establishes its location before auscultation (Fig. 2).

Auscultatory measurement of systolic and diastolic pressures

The stethoscope should be placed gently over the brachial artery at the point of maximal pulsation. A bell end-piece gives better sound reproduction but for in clinical practice a diaphragm is easier to secure with the fingers of one hand and covers a larger area. The stethoscope should be held firmly and evenly but without excessive pressure. Too much pressure may distort the artery, producing sounds below diastolic pressure. To avoid friction sounds the stethoscope end-piece should not touch the clothing, cuff, or rubber tubes (Fig. 2).

The cuff should then be inflated rapidly to about 30 mmHg above the palpated systolic pressure and deflated at a rate of 2 to 3 mmHg per pulse beat (or per second) during which the auscultatory phenomena described below will be heard. When all sounds have disappeared the cuff should be deflated rapidly and completely before repeating the measurement to prevent venous congestion of the arm. The following phases, first described by Nicolai Korotkov, may now be heard:

KOROTKOV PHASES

* Phase I – The first appearance of faint, repetitive, clear tapping sounds which gradually increase in intensity for at least two consecutive beats is the systolic blood pressure.

* Phase II – A brief period may follow during which the sounds soften and acquire a swishing quality.

* Phase III – The return of sharper sounds, which become crisper but never fully regain the intensity of phase I sounds. The clinical significance, if any, phases II and III has not been established.

* Phase IV – The distinct abrupt muffling of sounds, which become soft and blowing in quality.

* Phase V – The point at which all sounds finally disappear completely is the diastolic pressure.

Diastolic dilemma

Recommendations on blood pressure measurement have vacillated for many years on the issue of the diastolic end-point – the so-called diastolic dilemma. Phase IV (muffling) may coincide with or be as much as 10 mmHg higher than Phase V (disappearance), but usually the difference is less than 5 mmHg. Phase V correlates best with intra-arterial pressure, but general acceptance of the silent end-point has been resisted until recently because, in some groups of patients, for example in children, pregnant women, anaemic or elderly patients, the silent end-point may be greatly below the muffling of sounds. In some patients sounds may be audible when cuff pressure is deflated even to zero. The arguments for and against selecting one phase over the other have been well summarised but there is now a general concensus that disappearance of sounds (Phase V) should be taken as diastolic pressure except in pregnancy when disappearance of sounds may be greatly below muffling and in those patients in whom sounds persist down to zero.

Recording blood pressure

The blood pressure should be written down as soon as it has been recorded. Measurements of systolic and diastolic pressure should be made to the nearest 2 mmHg and rounding off to the nearest 5 or 10 mmHg (digit preference) is not permissible. The arm in which the pressure is being recorded and the position of the subject should be denoted and, on the first attendance, pressures should be recorded in both arms. In obese patients the bladder size should be indicated. If, as so often happens in practice, the observer has to make do with a 'standard' cuff containing a bladder with the dimensions 23 × 12 cm, it is best to state that measurement was made with such a cuff so that the presence of 'cuff hypertension' can be taken into account in diagnostic and management decisions and so that arrangements can be made for a more accurate measurement of blood pressure. In clinical practice the diastolic pressure should be recorded as Phase V except in those patients in whom sounds persist greatly below muffling and in pregnant women, in whom Phase IV should be recorded, but this should be clearly indicated. In hypertension research we recommend that both Phase IV and V be recorded. If the patient is so anxious, restless or distressed as to influence blood pressure behaviour, this should be recorded with the blood pressure. The presence of an auscultatory gap should always be indicated.

Finally, in patients taking blood pressure-lowering drugs the optimum time for measuring control of blood pressure will depend on the time of day at which the drugs are taken. It may be helpful, therefore, when assessing the effect of antihypertensive drugs, to note the time of drug ingestion in relation to the time of measurement.

KEY POINTS IN MEASURING BLOOD PRESSURE

* Have the subject seated comfortably

* Check the sphygmomanometer
  (meniscus at zero, tubing airtight, etc.)

* Remove restrictive clothes from arm

* Make sure bladder is of adequate length

* Apply cuff snugly
  (lower edge 2–3 cm above fossa)

* Palpate brachial artery pulsation

* Inflate cuff above disappearance of pulse

* Deflate cuff slowly and note point of reappearance of pulse

* Place stethoscope gently over point of maximal pulsation

* Inflate cuff to 30 mmHg above palpated systolic pressure

* Reduce pressure at rate of 2–3 mmHg per beat or per second

* Take reading of systolic pressure when repetitive, clear tapping sounds appear for two consecutive beats

* Take reading of diastolic pressure when repetitive sounds disappear

* Write down measurement immediately

A comprehensive recording of blood pressure in two clinical situations might, therefore, appear as follows:

First assessment – R arm 154/82; L arm 148/76; 35 cm bladder; sitting; subject anxious.

First assessment – R arm 210/52; L arm 204/48 (phase IV/auscultatory gap); 35 cm bladder; lying; 182/60 standing; medication at 8.00 hours/BP at 9.30 hours.

Number of measurements

It is recommended that one measurement be taken carefully at each visit, repeating the measurement if there is uncertainty or distraction, rather than making a number of hurried measurements. In patients in whom sustained increases of blood pressure are being assessed, a number of measurements should be made on different occasions over a number of weeks or months before diagnostic or management decisions are made.

Obtaining a blood pressure profile

Accurate though measurement may be when the above recommendations are followed, it should be realised that any such measurement represents only a fraction of the 24-hour blood pressure profile. Therefore, it is becoming common in clinical practice to obtain a profile of blood pressure over time before making decisions on diagnosis and treatment. The two most popular techniques are self-measurement and ambulatory measurement, though repeated measurements may give some indication of blood pressure behaviour.

OBTAINING A PROFILE OF BLOOD PRESSURE

Self (home) measurement

Since Brown's observation in 1930 that blood pressure measured in the home was lower than that recorded by a doctor, the discrepancy between pressures recorded in the home and the clinic has been repeatedly confirmed – as has the considerable individual variability. Assessed against clinic measurements blood pressure recorded at home is accurate whether measured by patients or their relatives or friends, and the technique can detect small average changes in blood pressure.

Why then has home measurement of blood pressure failed to achieve the popularity of home urinalysis in diabetes? There are a number of explanations. First, there is the problem of training the patient to measure blood pressure, though in our experience a satisfactory degree of competence can usually be achieved by using illustrated instructions; a further difficulty, which cannot easily be corrected, is that of subjective bias; the physician may be concerned about causing anxiety or causing the patient to take an obsessional interest in his or her blood pressure, and, finally, most devices available for self-measurement of blood pressure have not been validated adequately or have been shown to be inaccurate. For these reasons home measurement of blood pressure has not received widespread acceptance, though it has a useful place in carefully selected patients. Moreover, 24-hour ambulatory blood pressure measurement, by providing a more objective blood pressure profile during both day and night and also being free of bias, is becoming the preferred method of assessing blood pressure behaviour.

Ambulatory blood pressure measurement

Ambulatory blood pressure measurement over 24 hours has given new insights into blood pressure behaviour and is bringing about a reappraisal of previously held concepts of hypertension. The technique is rapidly gaining acceptance as a useful procedure in the clinical management of hypertension, in the assessment of antihypertensive drugs, and as a means of predicting outcome in hypertension.

Ambulatory blood pressure recording may prove to be one of the most significant developments in the clinical management of hypertension. The technique also has considerable potential in hypertension research. Undoubtedly its greatest value is the facility to assess blood pressure behaviour over a 24- or 48-hour period in the patient's own working and home environment. Data from ambulatory measurement suggests that many subjects are diagnosed, labelled and treated as hypertensive with conventional measurement who might not be so diagnosed by ambulatory blood pressure measurement. It has been estimated that as many as one fifth of patients diagnosed as hypertensive may be incorrectly diagnosed and inappropriately treated. Translated into fiscal terms this could represent an over-expenditure on antihypertensive drugs in the region of 5 billion dollars annually in the United States. Ambulatory blood pressure measurement, moreover, by providing a 24-hour profile of blood pressure, facilitates the prescribing of antihypertensive medication to suit the requirements of the individual patient and further reduces the cost of medication.

The increasing use of 24-hour ambulatory blood pressure measurement in clinical practice has shown a number of patterns of blood pressure behaviour, such as the 'white coat' effect whereby the circumstances of measurement may in themselves induce a rise in blood pressure.

BLOOD PRESSURE MEASUREMENT IN SPECIAL CIRCUMSTANCES

Obesity

The association between obesity and hypertension has been confirmed in many epidemiological studies and has at least two components. First, there appears to be a pathophysiological connection and it may well be that in some cases the two conditions are causally linked. The second is more pertinent to the present context in that obesity, if not taken into account, may result in inaccurate blood pressure values being obtained by inaccurate measurement techniques. The relationship between arm circumference and bladder dimension has been discussed above.

Arrhythmias

The major source of difficulty in blood pressure measurement when arrhythmias are present is the large variation in blood pressure from beat to beat when cardiac rhythm is irregular. Thus in arrhythmias, such as atrial fibrillation, stroke volume and as a consequence blood pressure, varies depending on the preceding pulse interval. Secondly, in such circumstances, there is no generally accepted method of determining auscultatory end-points. The lack of a uniform approach is reflected by the greater inter-observer variability when blood pressure is measured in atrial fibrillation than in sinus rhythm.

In bradyarrhythmias there may be two sources of error. First if the rhythm is irregular there will be the same problems as with atrial fibrillation. Secondly when the heart rate is extremely slow, for example 40 beats per minute, it is important that the deflation rate used is less than for normal heart rates as too-rapid deflation will lead to underestimation of systolic and overestimation of diastolic pressure.

Children

Blood pressure measurement in children presents a number of difficulties. Blood pressure variability is greater than in adults and thus any one reading is less likely to represent the true blood pressure in children. Also increased variability confers a greater tendency for regression towards the mean. Conventional sphygmomanometry is recommended for general use but systolic pressure is preferred to diastolic because of greater accuracy and reproducibility. Cuff dimensions are most important and three cuffs with bladders measuring 4 × 13 cm, 8 × 18 cm and the adult dimension 12 × 35 cm are required for the range of arm sizes likely to be encountered in the age range 0–14 years. The widest cuff practicable should be used. Korotkov sounds are not reliably audible in all children under one year and in many under five years of age. In such cases conventional sphygmomanometry is impossible and more sensitive methods of detection such as doppler, ultrasound or oscillometry must be used.

Pregnancy

Between 2 and 5% of pregnancies in Western Europe are complicated by clinically relevant hypertension and in a significant number of these the raised blood pressure is a key factor in medical decision making in the pregnancy. Particular attention must be paid to blood pressure measurement in pregnancy because of the important implications for patient management as well as the fact that blood pressure measurement in pregnancy presents some special problems.

As with essential hypertension and normotensives there are discrepancies between intra-arterial blood pressure values and those obtained by indirect measurement. However, it appears that this is not sufficient to invalidate decisions made on the basis of conventional clinical measurement.

Blood pressure levels are markedly affected by body position, particularly in the third trimester. Both systolic and diastolic pressures are about 10 mmHg lower in the left lateral recumbent position than in the sitting, supine and erect positions. Despite the documented importance of maternal position and the considerable differences between Phase IV and V in pregnancy there is considerable variation in the practice employed to measure blood pressure. Various positions are used and there is even lack of agreement as to the Korotkov phase for diastolic blood pressure, though Phase V is generally recommended.

Elderly

Blood pressure as measured in epidemiological and interventional studies predicts morbidity and mortality in the elderly as effectively as in the young.

The extent to which blood pressure conventionally measured predicts outcome may be influenced, not only by the strength of the association between raised blood pressure and outcome but also on various factors that influence the accuracy of blood pressure measurement and the extent to which casual blood pressure represents the blood pressure load on the heart and circulation.

Inaccuracy of the technique of measurement may result in blood pressure values being found that are at variance with the true blood pressure at the time of measurement and increased variability may affect the likelihood of a reading(s) being representative of blood pressure over time.

Of the pathophysiological changes that characterise hypertension in the elderly none is more apparent than the tendency to have raised systolic blood pressure and this finds its extreme form in isolated systolic hypertension. There is a decrease in the elasticity and distensibility of the ageing blood vessels due to changes in smooth muscle proliferation and alterations in elastin, collagen and calcium content leading to a decrease in compliance. One consequence of this is the increase in systolic blood pressure found in elderly hypertensives. A second consequence is that the decrease in compliance may interfere with the accuracy of indirect sphygmomanometry in the elderly. Indirect blood pressure measurement may overestimate blood pressure in the elderly. The term 'pseudohypertension' may be differentiated by the use of Osler's manoeuvre. William Osler observed that if after a blood pressure cuff is inflated above systolic pressure the artery remains palpable distal to the cuff the vessel is likely to be sclerosed. Patients in whom Osler's sign is positive have stiff arteries and a greater degree of 'pseudohypertension'.

Our studies have led us to conclude that the standard technique for blood pressure measurement with a mercury sphygmomanometer is as accurate in the elderly as in young patients in general. However, that is not to say that there are not some elderly hypertensive patients, prevalence unknown, who have a large disparity between direct and indirect blood pressure measurement and in such circumstances conventional sphygmomanometry may overestimate both systolic and diastolic blood pressure.

As blood pressure variability is increased in the elderly, blood pressure measurement is even less reliable in the older patient. Therefore the likelihood of any one reading being representative of blood pressure in general diminishes. To a greater or lesser extent this problem pertains in all patients due to various sources of variability including diurnal patterns, white coat effect, anxiety, cold, etc. One way of reducing the impact of the increased variability is to carry out repeated measurements, and this approach is particularly important in evaluating elderly patients.

Two extreme forms of blood pressure change which in the elderly are postural hypotension and postprandial hypotension. It is possible for postural hypotension to coexist with raised supine and sitting blood pressure and it is important that blood pressure is assessed in these positions, as well as standing, on initial assessment and subsequently from time to time if drugs known to cause postural hypotension are being taken. These include not only blood pressure-lowering drugs, such as diuretics, but also non-cardiovascular drugs, for example, neuroleptics and tricyclic antidepressants. Elderly patients get quite a marked blood pressure fall after eating and this may be symptomatic. Again this can only be diagnosed definitively by measuring blood pressure when standing after a meal.

Blood pressure measurement in critical care units

Complex devices that record blood pressure automatically at preset intervals have been designed for intensive care units and theatres. These devices often use two methods of measurement, most commonly Korotkov sound detection and oscillometry, but often the mode being used is not indicated and assessments of accuracy for each mode are sometimes not available from the manufacturers. Moreover, these devices do not always lend themselves to independent assessment because of their complex design.

Blood pressure measurement in research

Blood pressure measurement by an observer using a standard mercury sphygmomanometer and stethoscope is subject to observer prejudice and terminal digit preference. These limitations can introduce error which is unacceptable for research work. However, careful training of observers as described above can greatly reduce the error. Two devices have been designed specifically for research use – the random zero sphygmomanometer, which reduces observer prejudice, and the London School of Hygiene sphygmomanometer, which reduces both observer prejudice and terminal digit preference.

London School of Hygiene sphygmomanometer

This was the first such device to be introduced. By means of a series of columns and plungers the observer records pressure by depressing the appropriate plunger at the end-points for systolic pressure and phase IV and

V diastolic pressure without having any means of knowing the pressure in the cuff. Rather surprisingly the London School of Hygiene Sphygmomanometer was accepted as the 'gold standard' for blood pressure measurement without being subjected to validation. In 1982 a calibration error was demonstrated in the device which, as far as we know, has not been rectified by the manufacturers and the London School of Hygiene Sphygmomanometer is not now much used.

Random-zero sphygmomanometer

In 1963, Garrow described a 'zero-muddler for unprejudiced sphygmo-manometry' which was modified by Wright and Dore in 1970 and produced commercially by Messrs Hawksley and Sons. It is larger than a conventional sphygmomanometer and some ten times more expensive. The manometer function is similar to that of the mercury sphygmomanometer but a wheel is spun before each measurement to adjust the zero to an unknown level. Once the blood pressure has been measured the level of zero may be determined and the pressure reading corrected. In this way observer prejudice is reduced but not digit preference. This device is generally accepted as the instrument of choice for epidemiological and research studies because it reduces observer bias and obscures digit preference, though the facility of the device to reduce terminal digit preference has been questioned. Because the random-zero sphygmomanometer is basically a mercury sphygmomanometer, its accuracy has been accepted rather uncritically and it has replaced the London School of Hygiene Sphygmomanometer as the 'gold standard' against which other devices are assessed. However, recently it has been shown to systematically underestimate blood pressure, especially diastolic pressure and we have confirmed this tendency thus raising the question as to its suitability for research and epidemiological studies.

CONCLUDING COMMENT

For the future, careful measurement of blood pressure with a mercury sphygmomanometer following the above recommendations is likely to remain the most effective first line in assessing blood pressure. If conventional measurement is below 150/90 mmHg, especially over a number of measurements, that individual may be passed as normotensive. If, however, blood pressure is elevated above this level an assessment of blood pressure behaviour is helpful before making diagnostic and therapeutic decisions.

Selected references

Burke MJ, Tower H, O'Malley K, Fitzgerald DJ, O'Brien ET (1982): Sphygmomanometers in hospital and family practice: problems and recommendations. *Br Med J* 285: 469–471.

British Standards Institution (1990): Specification for aneroid and mercury non-automated sphygmomanometers (Revision of BS 2743: 1956 and BS 2744: 1956). British Standards Institution. London. In press.

Evans CE, Haynes RB, Goldsmith CH, Hewson SA (1989): Home blood pressure-measuring devices: a comparative study of accuracy. *J Hypertension* 7: 133–142.

Frohlich ED, Grim C, Labarthe DR, Maxwell MH, Perloff D, Weidman WH (1990): Report of a Special Task Force Appointed by the Steering Committee, American Heart Association. Recommendations for the human blood pressure determination by sphygmomanometers. *Circulation* [In press].

Manning DM, Kuchirka C, Kaminski J (1983): Miscuffing: inappropriate blood pressure cuff application. *Circulation* 68:763–766.

O'Brien E, O'Malley K (1987): The observer, the sphygmomanometer, the patient, technique, infancy and childhood, future trends. In: *ABC of Hypertension*. 2nd ed. British Medical Association. London.

O'Brien E, O'Malley K (1981): *Essentials of Blood Pressure Measurement*. Churchill Livingstone. Edinburgh, London, Melbourne & New York.

Parr GD, Poole PH (1988): Effects of sphygmomanometer type and position of the arm on blood pressure measurement. *J Hum Hypertension* 2: 153–156.

Petrie JC, O'Brien ET, Littler WA, de Swiet M (1986): Recommendations on blood pressure measurement. British Hypertension Society. *Br Med J* 293: 611–615.

Rose GA, Holland WW, Crowley EA (1964): A sphygmomanometer for epidemiologists. *Lancet* 1:296–300.

Short D (1976): The diastolic dilemma. *Br Med J* 2: 685–686.

Wilcox J (1961): Observer factors in the measurement of blood pressure. *Nurs Res* 10: 4–17.

CHAPTER 2

Pathophysiological basis of hypertension

ARMIN DISTLER and HERMANN HALLER

The two most important factors which determine the mean arterial blood pressure (MAP) in the systemic circulation are cardiac output (CO) and total peripheral vascular resistance (TPR), so that:

$$MAP = CO \times TPR$$

In most forms of hypertension systolic *and* diastolic blood pressures are increased. An elevated diastolic blood pressure is predominantly the consequence of an increased total peripheral vascular resistance. Isolated *systolic hypertension* may be caused by an increased cardiac output, e.g. in hyperthyroidism, or by an increased rigidity of the aorta, as occurs in the elderly.

In this chapter we intend to summarize various aspects of the pathophysiology of systolic and diastolic hypertension:

FACTORS IN HYPERTENSION

Essential hypertension

* Genetics
* Salt intake
* Cellular sodium/calcium transport
* Renal mechanisms
* Obesity, insulin resistance
* Renin–angiotensin-aldosterone and atrial natriuretic peptide
* Sympathetic nervous system
* Stress
* Structural alterations

Secondary hypertension

* Renal parenchymatous disease
* Renal artery stenosis
* Endocrine causes
* Aortic coarctation
* Drugs

ESSENTIAL HYPERTENSION

The diagnosis of 'essential hypertension' is made after secondary forms of hypertension have been ruled out. Essential hypertension is a heterogeneous disease whose aetiology is only partially understood. A series of factors are known to favour the manifestation of essential hypertension (Fig.1) none of which probably plays a dominating role. Rather the main disturbance appears to be an inappropriate interplay of the various factors responsible for normal blood pressure regulation. This does not preclude that a distinct factor such as a high salt intake in a salt-sensitive subject or obesity may play a dominant role in a given patient. In the early stages of essential hypertension the cardiac output is often slightly elevated whereas the total peripheral resistance is still normal. This results in a mild blood pressure elevation since total peripheral vascular resistance is not decreased appropriately in relation to the increased cardiac output. These changes are probably caused by an increased adrenergic activity. Blood volume may be decreasesd while cardiopulmonary blood volume tends to be normal. As the disease progresses the total peripheral vascular resistance increases. The hallmark of established hypertension is an increased total peripheral resistance. The increase in vascular resistance is caused by vasoconstriction and/or by a structural narrowing of the vascular lumen of the precapillary resistance vessels, mainly in the splanchnic and renal vascular bed (see Structural Alterations).

GENETICS OF ESSENTIAL HYPERTENSION

Hypertension tends to aggregate within families. On the average, the relatives of hypertensives have higher blood pressure levels at all ages than the relatives of normotensive subjects. Persons with a family history of hypertension are about twice as likely to become hypertensive than those with a negative family history. From studies of hypertensive families, it has been estimated that about 20% of the diastolic blood pressure variance and 33% of the systolic blood pressure variance are determined by genetic factors. The level of blood pressure is continuously distributed within a given population (so-called unimodal distribution) i.e. there is no sharp dividing line between normotensive and hypertensive blood pressure levels. Obviously no single pattern of inheritance can explain this unimodal distribution of blood pressure, making mutations at different gene loci i.e. polygeneity the most likely mode of inheritance. The question remains: which are the genetic defects transmitted by the multiple genes involved? Genetic defects may affect renal mechanisms (see Salt and Hypertension and Kidney and Hypertension), cell membrane alterations (see Disturbances of Cellular Transport),

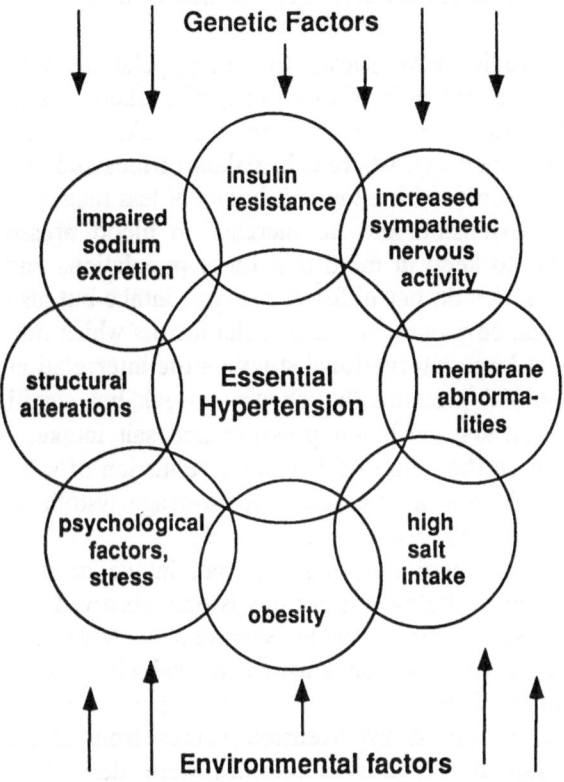

Fig. 1. Genetic influence and environmental factors in the development of essential hypertension

humoral factors (see Insulin and Hypertension) or neural mechanisms (see Stress and Hypertension).

As already mentioned, it is unlikely that a single genetic defect will explain the pathogenesis of essential hypertension. Genetic heterogeneity of a common disease means different modes of inheritance, ethnic variability, and the association with a variety of genetic markers. It would therefore be necessary to characterize the dominant traits or to find marker genes for essential hypertension. In recent years, several investigators have demonstrated DNA polymorphisms in hypertensive rat strains. DNA polymorphisms were found for the renin gene, the NaK-ATPase gene and the kallikrein gene. However, a cosegregation of high blood pressure and DNA polymorphism has not yet been convincingly shown in hypertensive rat strains or in human essential hypertension.

SALT INTAKE AND HYPERTENSION (see also Chapter 7)

Epidemiological studies have shown that in populations with a high salt intake, i.e. in the western industrialized countries, there is a uniformly high prevalence of hypertension. The average salt intake in western countries amounts to 12–15 g per day, whereas in Eskimo tribes and in some isolated populations in the tropics with a low salt intake of less than 3 g daily, there is practically no hypertension and no increase in blood pressure with age. However, one has to keep in mind that these populations and the western industrialized countries do not differ only in salt intake but also with respect to other nutritional, environmental and social factors which may affect blood pressure. A recent large international study on the interrelationship between salt intake and blood pressure has shown a weak but significant positive correlation between systolic blood pressure and salt intake. According to calculations based on the data of this study a reduction of salt intake by 6 g per day would result in a diminuition of the average systolic blood pressure rise between the 25th and 35th year of 9 mm Hg.

A rise in blood pressure during high salt intake or a decrease upon restriction of salt intake below 6 g per day is only observed in about 40% of all patients with essential hypertension. Such patients have been classified as being salt sensitive. In most salt-sensitive individuals a familial history of hypertension can be demonstrated. Further evidence for a strong genetic background of salt-induced hypertension comes from selective breeding experiments in rats in which two colonies were derived from a single Sprague–Dawley strain. In one colony the rats rapidly developed hypertension (so-called 'Dahl S-rats' in which S is for sensitive) on the same high salt intake to which members of the other colony were resistant (so-called 'Dahl R-rats'). The blood pressure rise in the Dahl S-rats is probably the consequence of an inherited defect in renal sodium excretion.

The blood pressure-raising effect of salt is not only related to the Na^+ cation. Experimental studies both in the rat and in man have demonstrated that the Cl^- anion is also of importance since no blood pressure rise occurred when a sodium load was given as $NaHCO_3$ or a combination of sodium bicarbonate/phosphate/glycinate instead of NaCl.

DISTURBANCES OF CELLULAR SODIUM TRANSPORT

The precise mechanisms underlying salt sensitivity have not yet been fully elucidated. Several disturbances of cellular sodium transport mechanisms have been described in animal models of hypertension as well as in essential hypertension. It is uncertain, however, to what extent the effect of high salt intake on blood pressure is mediated through these mechanisms.

Intracellular sodium concentration

Several authors have described an increased sodium concentration in erythrocytes of patients with essential hypertension. This finding has, however, been questioned by others. More consistently, an elevated sodium concentration has been found in leukocytes of patients with essential hypertension. It is still unclear whether the increased intracellular sodium is predominantly due to a decreased maximal Na^+-pump activity, an increased Na^+–H^+ exchange or to an increased Na^+ influx.

Na^+-pump activity (Na^+–K^+-ATPase)

A lower maximal velocity (V_{max}) of Na^+–K^+-ATPase (which serves as a sodium pump) has repeatedly been found in erythrocytes and lymphocytes of patients with essential hypertension (Fig. 2). The decreased pump activity has been attributed to a circulating inhibitor of the Na^+–K^+-ATPase (the 'natriuretic hormone'). This putative factor is presumed to be secreted by the hypothalamus and is stimulated by increased salt intake and/or by volume expansion. An inhibition, by this factor, of the Na^+–K^+-ATPase in the kidneys would result in an increased tubular sodium reabsorption and, in the vascular smooth muscle cells, in an increased intracellular sodium concentration. The chemical nature of this factor is unknown so far. Since it has been bound to digitalis antibodies, a digitalis-like structure has been postulated.

Na^+–Li^+ countertransport

Erythrocytes show a countertransport system exchanging Na^+ for Li^+ at a ratio of 1:1 which can be examined by monitoring the rate of exchange of internal Li^+ for external Na^+– and has therefore been named Na^+–Li^+ countertransport. No obvious function is known for this transport system. An elevated V_{max} for the Na^+–Li^+ countertransport has been found in the erythrocytes of a substantial number of patients with essential hypertension as well as in offspring of hypertensives. It has been suggested that changes in membrane organization may contribute to the elevated V_{max} observed in hypertensives (see also below, Membrane Alterations in Essential Hypertension). However, the exact cause of the elevated V_{max} is still poorly understood.

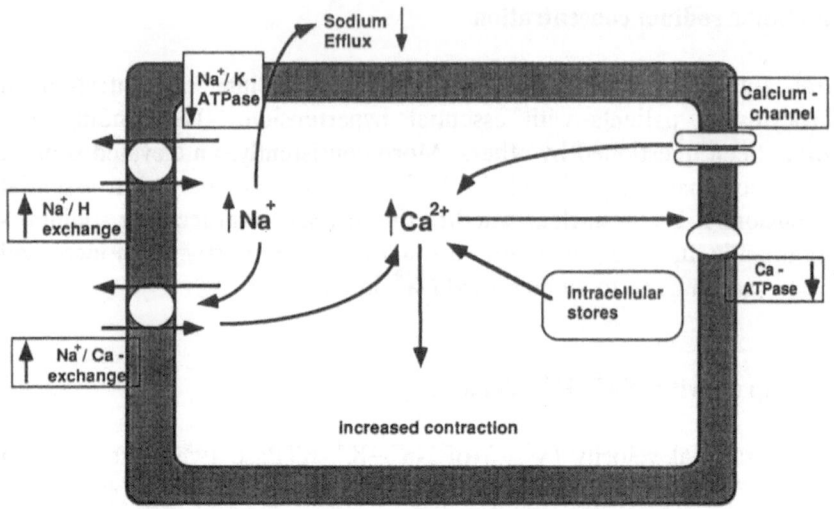

Fig. 2. Intracellular regulation of calcium and its possible relationship with sodium transport defects which have been found to be altered in patients with essential hypertension. An inhibition of the sodium pump (Na-K-ATPase) and/or an increased activity of the Na/H exchange mechanism would result in an increased intracellular free sodium concentration. The increased sodium concentration could be linked to the calcium regulation in the cell via the Na/Ca exchange mechanism. A high intracellular free calcium concentration in hypertension could also be due to an increased influx of calcium via the plasma membrane calcium channels or to a decrease in the calcium efflux due to a decreased activity of the calcium pump (Ca-ATPase)

Na$^+$–H$^+$ exchange

The Na$^+$–H$^+$ exchange is a ubiquitous transport pathway which is driven by the Na$^+$ and H$^+$ gradients across the cell membrane. In red blood cells of patients with essential hypertension and of spontaneously hypertensive rats, increased rates of Na$^+$–H$^+$ exchange have been observed. Provided that this phenomenon also took place in vascular smooth muscle cells and/or nerve terminals, a permanent elevation of sodium concentration would result (Fig. 3). In the renal proximal tubule, overactivity of the luminal membrane Na$^+$–H$^+$ exchange would enhance sodium reabsorption and lead to a decreased salt excretion.

Na–Ca exchange

The pathophysiological significance of an increased sodium concentration in blood cells and, possibly, vascular smooth muscle cells for vasoconstriction per se is not clear. However, according to a hypothesis by Blaustein, an increased intracellular sodium concentration would result in an increase in intracellular free calcium via a sodium–calcium exchange system. In several cell types, the existence of such a sodium–calcium transport system has been demonstrated which exchanges two sodium for three calcium ions. According to the Blaustein hypothesis the increase in intracellular free calcium would then be directly responsible for the increased vasoconstriction in essential hypertension (Fig. 2).

Intracellular calcium regulation

Intracellular free, i.e. cytosolic, calcium concentration is an important determinant of vascular smooth muscle tension. Over the last few years, it has been demonstrated that in a proportion of patients with essential hypertension, intracellular free calcium in platelets is elevated. The cause of the elevated intracellular free calcium concentration in smooth muscle cells and platelets could be: (i) an increased influx, e.g. via the sodium–calcium exchange, or an increased release of calcium from intracellular stores; (ii) a reduction in calcium efflux from the cell or decreased calcium uptake by the endoplasmic reticulum; or (iii) a decreased calcium buffering due to a decrease in calcium binding to proteins. In smooth muscle cells from spontaneously hypertensive rats and in blood cells from patients with essential hypertension, it has been shown that calcium efflux, i.e. the activity of the calcium ATPase, is reduced, and the release of calcium from intracellular stores is increased. The intracellular buffering of calcium by protein binding is also decreased, thereby contributing to the elevated intracellular free calcium.

Recently, it has been demonstrated that it is not only intracellular free calcium concentration but also calcium-dependent processes within the cell which are activated in essential hypertension. One of these mechanisms being activated is the calcium-dependent protein kinase C, which may be of importance not only in systemic vasoconstriction but also in the proliferative response of vascular smooth muscle cells.

Cell membrane alterations

An altered membrane lipid composition with an increase in sialic acid and a decrease in polyunsaturated fatty acids as well as a decrease in membrane fluidity has been described in red blood cells from patients with essential hypertension by several investigators.

31

It has been suggested that the altered composition of the cell membrane in essential hypertension might contribute to the subtle alterations of sodium transport and calcium handling which have been observed in patients with essential hypertension.

THE KIDNEY IN ESSENTIAL HYPERTENSION

The kidney plays an important role in normal blood pressure regulation and in the pathogenesis of high blood pressure in hypertensive disorders. It has been shown that transplantation of a kidney from a normotensive donor into a patient with end-stage renal failure due to nephrosclerosis can lead to remission of essential hypertension. In the Milan strain of hypertensive rats transplantation of a kidney from a normotensive rat also induces a fall in blood pressure. Conversely, if kidneys from stroke-prone spontaneously hypertensive rats are transplanted into normotensive animals these rats develop an increase in blood pressure.

Pressure–natriuresis relationship

Normally the kidney responds to elevation of blood pressure and increased perfusion of the kidney by an increase in sodium and water excretion. The resulting reduction in fluid volume serves to return elevated blood pressure levels to normal. Normal individuals with an increase in dietary salt intake need only a small increase in blood pressure to raise their sodium excretion (Fig. 3). In patients with essential hypertension the natriuresis occurs at a higher arterial pressure, i.e. the pressure–natriuresis relationship is shifted, although the slope is similar (in contrast to compromised renal function). A renal defect of sodium excretion has been considered to be of primary importance in the pathogenesis of essential hypertension. This hypothesis is supported by the fact that already in normotensive subjects with a family history of essential hypertension, a decreased response in renal sodium elimination could be demonstrated. (See also pp. 41–43.)

OBESITY, INSULIN RESISTANCE AND HYPERTENSION

Obesity is a well-known predisposing factor for hypertension and weight reduction leads to a fall in blood pressure in obese hypertensives. Body weight appears to have a greater impact on blood pressure in females than in males. The mechanisms involved are poorly understood. An increase in

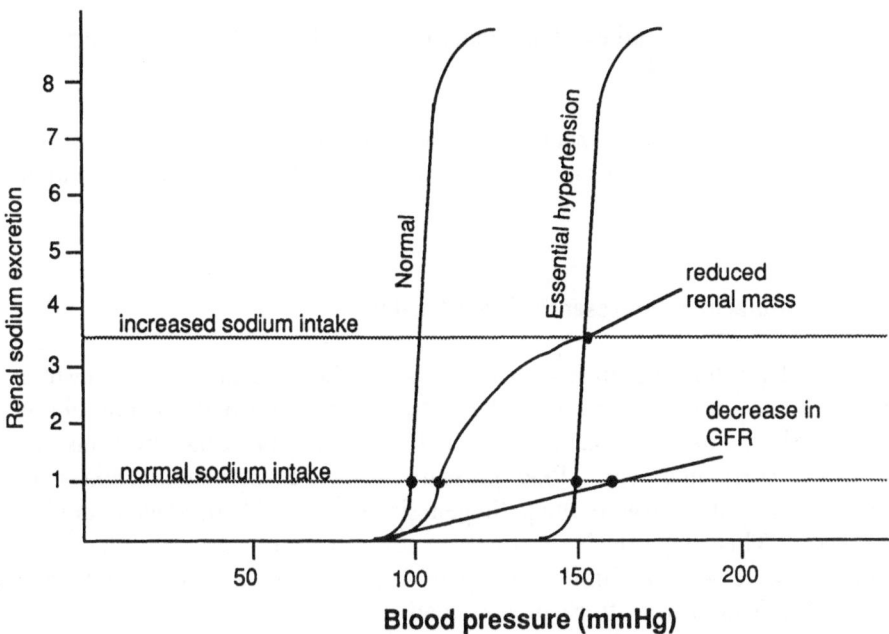

Fig. 3. Relationship between arterial pressure and sodium excretion with a normal and with a high-salt diet. The first curve shows the correlation between pressure and natriuresis in normal subjects. A high-salt diet in these subjects leads only to a small increase in blood pressure. In essential hypertension this correlation is not altered but the curve is shifted to raise a higher blood pressure level. If renal function is altered, e.g. a decrease in GFR or reduced renal mass, the necessary increase in blood pressure to maintain sodium excretion is much higher

cardiac output and high dietary salt intake, together with the high-calorie diet and an increased sympathetic nervous activity have been considered to be responsible for obesity-related hypertension.

Recently the well-documented hyperinsulinaemia of obese subjects has been related to the pathogenesis of the increased blood pressure. The hyperinsulinaemia seems to be due, besides diet and diminished hepatic insulin extraction, to a relative insulin resistance of peripheral tissue. Skeletal muscle and adipose tissue of such patients show a decreased sensitivity to insulin-mediated glucose uptake. The insulin resistance seems to be a 'post-receptor defect' of the insulin receptor in these tissues and is comparable to the defect observed in diabetes mellitus type II (non-insulin-dependent diabetes mellitus). The high insulin plasma levels may lead to an increase in blood pressure in two ways:

1. High plasma levels of insulin lead to increased plasma concentrations of noradrenaline. This effect is not due to a direct effect of insulin on

33

peripheral nerve endings but seems rather to be mediated by effects of insulin on the CNS.

2. High levels of plasma insulin have an antinatriuretic effect by increasing the sodium reabsorption in the distal tubule, thus leading to sodium retention.

Hyperinsulinaemia and essential hypertension

Peripheral insulin resistance associated with higher plasma levels of insulin following an oral glucose load has also been described in non-obese hypertensives and it has been shown that insulin plasma concentrations are positively correlated with blood pressure levels. Hyperinsulinaemia may therefore also play a role in the pathogenesis of essential hypertension in lean subjects. This hypothesis is further supported by the findings that normotensives with a family history of hypertension also display higher plasma levels of insulin after a glucose load.

Insulin resistance and hyperinsulinaemia in hypertensive patients may also be related to abnormalities of the lipoprotein metabolism, i.e. increased very-low density lipoproteins (VLDL) and decreased high-density lipoproteins are frequently observed in patients with essential hypertension. It has therefore been suggested that insulin resistance, hyperinsulinaemia, high plasma levels of VLDL and hypertension occur together as symptoms of a common syndrome, which has been called syndrome X, the common link being the peripheral insulin resistance. This syndrome may be of great importance in the pathogenesis of atherosclerosis and, in particular, coronary artery disease (see also Chapter 3).

THE RENIN–ANGIOTENSIN–ALDOSTERONE SYSTEM (RAAS) AND ATRIAL NATRIURETIC PEPTIDE (ANP)

The renin–angiotensin–aldosterone system is an important part of the physiological mechanism for blood pressure homoeostasis. The activity of the RAAS, as judged from plasma renin activity, is elevated only in about 15% of patients with essential hypertension. In these patients the increased plasma levels of angiotensin II could directly contribute to the increased vascular tone. The cause of the increased renin secretion by the juxtaglomerular cells in these patients could be an increased sympathetic tone or a decreased renal perfusion due to either increased afferent arteriolar resistance (in younger patients) or nephrosclerosis.

In most patients with essential hypertension plasma renin activity is within normal limits. However, because high blood pressure normally suppresses renin secretion the 'normal' plasma renin values in these patients are high in relation to their blood pressure. These 'inappropriately' normal renin levels may give an explanation for why ACE-inhibitors still induce a fall in blood pressure in those patients in whom the plasma renin activity is not elevated.

A second possible role of the RAAS in essential hypertension is a disturbance in the finely tuned interaction between renin secretion and sodium balance. Hypertensive patients have an abnormally wide variance of renin activity in relation to their sodium excretion. It has therefore been suggested that hypertensives can be classified as 'low-renin' or 'high-renin' hypertensives. As already mentioned, 15% of hypertensive patients have an elevated plasma renin activity while 25% of the hypertensive population are 'low-renin' hypertensives. It has been suggested that high renin plasma levels in hypertensive patients directly reflect the renin-mediated vasoconstriction. These patients are also relatively volume depleted. Patients with low renin plasma levels, on the other hand, are thought (although not proven) to have an increased extracellular volume due to increased sodium reabsorption. High- and low-renin hypertensives might therefore represent the two extremes of renin dependency vs sodium dependency of hypertension.

Over the last years local RAAS in different tissues (e.g. in the brain, in the heart or in the vessel wall) have been identified and their significance in cardiovascular regulation is a subject of intensive research.

Atrial natriuretic peptide (ANP)

This hormone is secreted from the atria of the heart in response to volume overload and an increase in atrial pressure. ANP leads to vasodilatation and natriuresis. In contrast to the postulated natriuretic hormone (see above) ANP does not inhibit the sodium pump but rather exerts its effects through cGMP. There is no good evidence that ANP is involved in the pathogenesis of essential hypertension. In most patients with essential hypertension the plasma concentrations of the hormone are within the normal range. In more severe hypertension circulating plasma levels of ANP are elevated, most probably due to a rise in atrial pressure.

THE SYMPATHETIC NERVOUS SYSTEM IN ESSENTIAL HYPERTENSION

An increase in sympathetic activity leads to the release of noradrenaline from sympathetic nerve endings, and adrenaline, from the adrenal medulla. An increased activity of the sympathetic nervous system has repeatedly been incriminated in the pathogenesis of essential hypertension. Indirect evidence for a role of the sympathetic nervous system in hypertension comes from the blood pressure-lowering effect of drugs which interfere with the sympathetic nervous system in patients with essential hypertension, such as α-methyldopa or clonidine. The increased cardiac output in young hypertensives has also been linked to an increased sympathetic drive in these patients.

An increased sympathetic activity in essential hypertension could be due to:

- an increased sympathetic outflow,
- a decrease in the reuptake of noradrenaline into intracellular storage sites, or
- an altered intracellular metabolism of noradrenaline (Fig. 4).

In addition, the effect of the catecholamines is also determined by the responsiveness of these organs, i.e. the number and affinity of postsynaptic receptors as well as the activity of intracellular messenger systems.

Plasma catecholamines

As it is hardly possible to directly evaluate the sympathetic activity by measuring the action potential in sympathetic nerve endings or the release of noradrenaline into the synaptic cleft, an indirect approach to investigation sympathetic nervous activity has been to measure plasma concentrations and urinary excretion of catecholamines. Such measurements are based on the assumption that increased sympathetic activity leads to an overflow of noradrenaline from the synaptic cleft into the blood. Plasma noradrenaline concentrations, thought to reflect sympathetic nervous activity, have been found to be elevated in patients with essential hypertension by 25% on average with considerable overlap of the values in hypertensives and normotensives. Such increases may also be found in patients with normal blood pressure, e.g. in patients with endogenous depression or with hypothyroidism. Therefore, an increased sympathetic tone can only be considered to be meaningful for blood pressure elevation if the pressor response to the sympathetic neurotransmitter, noradrenaline, is similarly

36

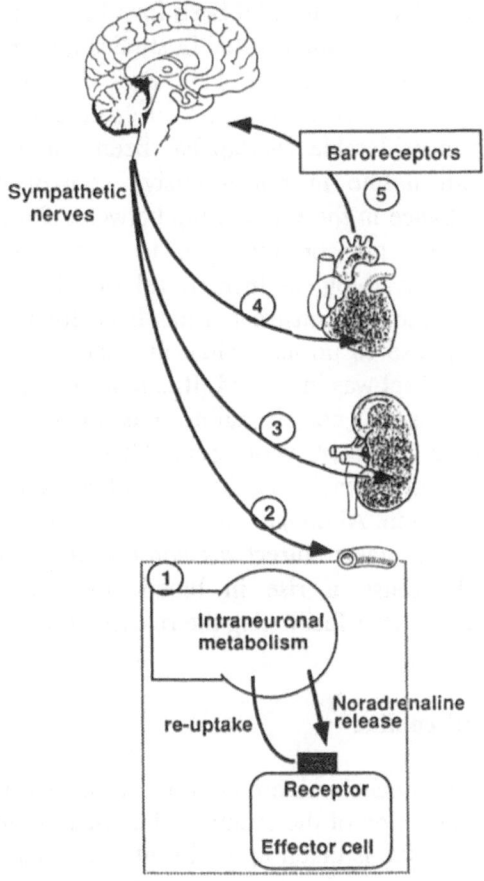

(1) altered intraneuronal metabolism of noradrenalin

(2) increased secretion of noradrenaline into the synaptic cleft

(3) increased stimulation of renal sympathetic nerves

(4) increased sympathetic drive

(5) resetting of the baroreceptors

Fig. 4. Scheme of the blood pressure regulatory mechanisms of the autonomous nervous system. An increase in sympathetic outflow from the brain can influence circulatory blood pressure via (1) an increased release of noradrenaline into the synaptic cleft or an altered intraneuronal metabolism of the catecholamines, (2) an increase in peripheral vasoconstriction, (3) increased sodium reabsorption in the renal tubules and/or a stimulatory effect on the adrenals, and (4) increased sympathetic stimulation of the heart. A decrease in the sensitivity of the baroreceptor (5) attenuates the cardiovascular reflexes and results in an additional increase in mean arterial blood pressure

increased. In fact, an increased pressor response to exogenous noradrenaline has repeatedly (although not uniformly) been found in patients with essential hypertension. This has been demonstrated in studies on forearm blood flow, and the reactivity of the capillary bed of the digit or nailfold, as well as in studies on the effects of intravenous noradrenaline on systemic blood pressure. Again, a considerable overlap has been found with the pressor responses to noradrenaline in normotensive control subjects. More consistently, a disturbance in the relationship between plasma noradrenaline concentration and the pressor response to noradrenaline has been demonstrated. The physiological inverse relationship between plasma noradrenaline and pressor responsiveness has been found to be shifted so that the pressor response to noradrenaline in relation to the concomitant plasma noradrenaline level was increased. It is noteworthy that an increased pressor responsiveness to noradrenaline has also been observed in normotensive offspring of patients with essential hypertension.

Increased plasma adrenaline levels have also been observed in patients with essential hypertension. Although adrenaline, at concentrations observed in essential hypertension, has no direct vasoconstrictor effect, such increased concentrations could cause a rise in blood pressure by acting upon presynaptic β_2-receptors, thus facilitating the release of noradrenaline.

Metabolism of noradrenaline

The measurement of catecholamine concentration in peripheral blood may not be an accurate reflection of the events in the synaptic cleft, since most of the noradrenaline released is taken up again into intracellular storage sites. The removal of noradrenaline has been shown to be slower in patients with essential hypertension. The reduced clearance of noradrenaline may be due to a decline in neuronal reuptake or the intraneuronal metabolism of noradrenaline.

BARORECEPTOR REFLEXES

Blood pressure increases detected by the baroreceptors of the aortic arch and the carotid sinus normally increase vagal and reduce sympathetic nervous activity. The sensitivity of the baroreceptors decreases with older age and with high blood pressure due to structural vascular alterations. When arterial pressure rises the sensitivity of the baroreceptor decreases within several days and therefore represents a consequence rather than a cause of the hypertension. However, the lower sensitivity of the baroreceptors may allow, via a decrease in vagal activity or an increase in sympathetic tone, the blood pressure to rise further during psychological stress or physical exercise and may therefore contribute to the development and maintenance of hypertension.

STRESS AND HYPERTENSION

Psychological factors are likely to contribute to the development of hypertension. Subjects exposed to repeated psychogenic stress develop hypertension more frequently. For instance, air traffic controllers, who work under high stress, develop hypertension 6 times more frequently than do nonprofessional pilots. Individuals living in protected societies like nuns have been found to have low blood pressure which does not rise with aging. In hypertensives a lesser exposure to daily stressful situations like during hospital admission leads to a fall or even a normalization of blood pressure. Predisposed subjects may therefore become hypertensive because their reactions to the normal stress of daily life are exaggerated. Several authors have in fact observed that hypertensive patients show a greater cardiovascular reactivity to psychological stress.

STRUCTURAL ALTERATIONS IN ESSENTIAL HYPERTENSION

An increase in arterial blood pressure in humans as well as in animal studies leads, within a relatively short time, to a thickening of the media of arteries and arterioles. This thickening of the media is due mainly to hypertrophy of vascular smooth muscle cells. Later on, there is also an increase in extracellular matrix production. The increase of the medial layer of the vessel wall diminishes the inner diameter of the small arteries and arterioles, i.e. the wall–lumen ratio of the blood vessel increases. As arteriolar resistance changes with the fourth power of the inner radius, even a small narrowing in the diameter of the vessels leads to a considerable increase in peripheral resistance.

Furthermore, the response of the hypertrophied arterioles to hormonal and neural stimulation is significantly amplified compared with normal arterioles.

As the hypertrophy of the media is induced by the increase in blood pressure, it seems to be a result of high blood pressure rather than a cause of hypertension. However, *in vitro* it has been clearly demonstrated that vascular smooth muscle cells from prehypertensive animals show an increased proliferative response to vasoactive stimuli and growth factors, indicating a genetic basis for the vascular hypertrophy.

Cardiac hypertrophy

Cellular hypertrophy in essential hypertension is induced not only in the vascular wall but also, and perhaps even more so, in the myocardium. Already in the early stages of essential hypertension there is an increase in left-ventricular mass due to hypertrophy of the myocytes. Echocardiography has disclosed an increased wall thickness in about 30% of subjects with mild hypertension (and normal electrocardiograms). Even in subjects with borderline hypertension, the thickness of the intraventricular septum is frequently increased. This hypertrophy seems to be a functional response to the increased wall stress caused by raised afterload. The increase in wall stress is almost completely offset by the depth of thickening.

Myocardial hypertrophy is not just a simple consequence of high blood pressure, although there is some relationship between the duration of high blood pressure and the stage of hypertrophy.

In younger patients, especially, it is probably also due to an increased activity of myocardial sympathetic nerves or the local renin–angiotensin system.

As in the case of the hypertrophy of the vascular smooth muscle cells in hypertension it is also possible that genetic alterations of the myocytes, i.e. intrinsic cellular abnormalities of the myocardium contribute to the increased growth response of the myocytes.

SECONDARY FORMS OF HYPERTENSION

Many of the factors contributing to high blood pressure which have been discussed in the previous sections are effective in secondary forms of hypertension. Among these factors are heredity, media hypertrophy of the resistance vessels and diminished sensitivity of the baroreceptors.

HYPERTENSION ASSOCIATED WITH RENAL PARENCHYMATOUS DISEASE

The kidney plays a central role in the long-term regulation of normal as well as pathologically elevated blood pressure. In particular, the kidney can influence the blood pressure level via the following mechanisms:

KIDNEY AND BLOOD PRESSURE

* excretion of sodium chloride and water

* secretion of renin

* secretion of prostaglandins, kallikrein and kinins

Excretory renal function, the renin–angiotensin system and prostaglandin and kallikrein–kinin formation are functionally interconnected.

Disturbance of excretory renal function and hypertension

Hypertension can develop in any type of renal disease associated with an impairment of function. In bilateral renal parenchymatous diseases, there is a disturbed relationship between systemic pressure and natriuresis/diuresis (Fig. 3). An elevation of systemic blood pressure normally leads to increased excretion of sodium chloride and water thereby reducing the blood volume, the venous return to the heart and the cardiac output. In cases of bilateral renal damage, the relationship between pressure and natriuresis/diuresis is disturbed in such a way that an adequate excretion of sodium chloride and water is only ensured at higher pressures following an increase in cardiac output (see box on p. 42).

This sequence of haemodynamic changes first observed in dogs after reduction of the renal parenchyma by a 5/6 nephrectomy was basically confirmed in long-term investigations in patients with chronic glomerulonephritis. The mechanism of the increase in total peripheral resistance after initial elevation of cardiac output is still poorly understood. It has been attributed to 'autoregulation' of blood flow in response to overperfusion of the tissues in relation to metabolic needs.

SEQUENCE OF EVENTS FOLLOWING
BILATERAL RENAL DAMAGE

impairment of excretory renal function
↓
retention of sodium chloride and water
↓
increase in total exchangeable sodium and blood volume
↓
increase in venous return to the heart
↓
elevation of cardiac output
↓
rise in total peripheral resistance

Renin–angiotensin system

Increased renin secretion by the kidneys only takes place in part of the patients with renal parenchymatous hypertension. As mentioned above, total exchangeable sodium and blood volume tend to be increased in this group of patients. Since renin secretion is normally inversely related to the exchangeable sodium, blood volume and blood pressure, patients with diseases of the renal parenchyma would be expected to have decreased plasma renin and angiotensin II levels. Thus the normal angiotensin II concentrations observed in the majority of such patients must be regarded as elevated in proportion to exchangeable sodium, blood volume and blood pressure and thereby may contribute to the elevation of blood pressure. The significance of the renin–angiotensin system for the pathogenesis of hypertension also emerges from the observation that bilateral nephrectomy in patients with severe renal parenchymatous hypertension generally leads to a complete normalization of blood pressure, probably due to the cessation of renal renin formation.

Prostaglandin and kinin formation

It has been suggested that a decreased renal production of antihypertensive eicosanoids (e.g. PGE_2) or, less frequently, an increased production of prohypertensive eicosanoids (e.g. thromboxane) may contribute to the pathogenesis of renal hypertension. The relative combination of each of these factors varies with the hypertensive model and species so that no firm conclusion can be drawn about the role of eicosanoids in renal or other forms of hypertension.

The renal kallikrein–kinin system seems also to participate in blood pressure regulation in close relationship with the renin–angiotensin system, prostaglandins, the sympathetic nervous system and the control of electrolyte and water excretion. However, its precise role in the pathogenesis of renal or other forms of hypertension is still unclear.

RENOVASCULAR HYPERTENSION (See also Chapter 6)

Renovascular hypertension usually develops if one or several renal artery stenoses lead to underperfusion of one or both kidneys. Renovascular hypertension in humans corresponds to the animal model of hypertension that develops after clamping the blood flow of one or both renal arteries (so-called Goldblatt hypertension). The juxtaglomerular cells acting as baroreceptors react to the resulting pressure reduction by increasing formation and release of renin. However, the concentration of renin only increases in the ischaemic kidney and in the peripheral blood if there is an intact contralateral kidney. If the contralateral kidney has been removed, the hypertension produced by clamping the blood flow of the renal artery is usually even more severe than that in the presence of an intact contralateral kidney, but an increased renin release does not occur. Thus, two forms of experimental renal hypertension can be distinguished after the reduction of renal blood flow: one that is accompanied by an activation of the renin–angiotensin system and one in which the system is not stimulated.

The following will deal only with the present concepts regarding the pathophysiology of renovascular hypertension in the presence of an intact contralateral kidney (so-called 1C–2K (= 1 clip – 2 kidneys) hypertension) (see Fig. 5). This type of hypertension develops stepwise via the following mechanisms:

Phase 1: The blood pressure increase within minutes of constriction of a renal artery is very probably due to the direct pressor effect of angiotensin II.

Phase 2: Sodium and water retention develops as the result of a stimulation of aldosterone secretion, a reduced perfusion pressure in the clamped kidney and possibly also a direct tubular effect of angiotensin II. The sodium and water retention leads to a drop in the plasma concentrations of renin and angiotensin II. Within one week of constriction of a renal artery, the plasma concentrations of renin and angiotensin II tend to return to baseline levels, while hypertension continues or even increases. A further consequence of sodium and water retention is an increase in intravascular volume and thus also in cardiac output. In a later phase, there is an additional increase in the total peripheral resistance, the cause of which is not fully understood. Hypertension will recede again in this phase after removal of the stenosis.

Phase 3: Phase 3 is arbitrarily separated from phase 2 and designates the stage of renal hypertension in which elimination of the stenosis no longer leads to a decrease in blood pressure. At this stage, hypertension is maintained by the vascular and parenchymal damage caused by the increased blood pressure in the contralateral kidney. In this phase, the mechanisms of maintenance of hypertension thus correspond to those of renal–parenchymatous hypertension.

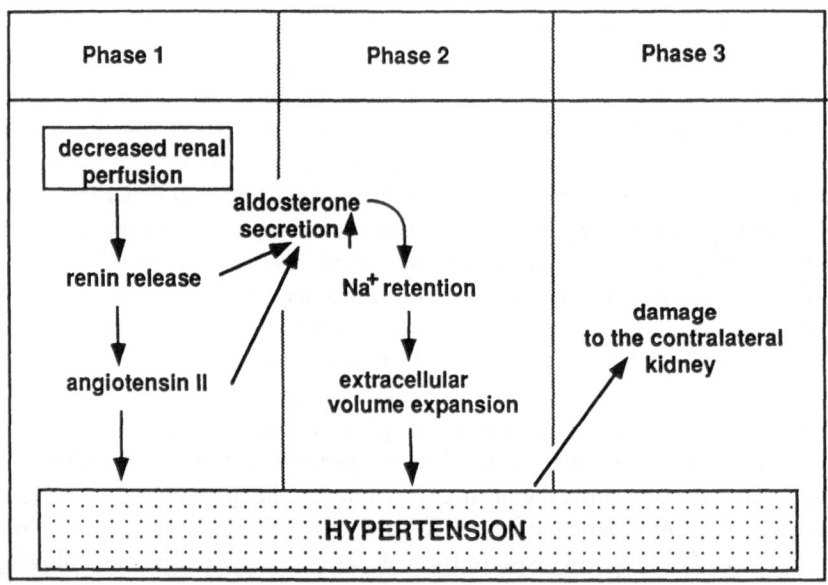

Fig.5. Stages in the development of renovascular hypertension

ENDOCRINE FORMS OF HYPERTENSION (See also Chapter 6)

Cushing's syndrome

The clinical symptoms of Cushing's syndrome are caused by increased cortisol secretion due to: enhanced ACTH formation by the pituitary (about

85%); an ectopic ACTH-producing tumour; or an adenoma or carcinoma (rare) of the adrenal cortex. Noteworthy is the fact that hypertension is observed in around 80% of patients with Cushing's syndrome but in only about 20% of those under chronic glucocorticoid therapy. The hypertensive mechanism of the glucocorticoids is largely unclarified. Findings obtained in animal experiments are limited in their applicability to hypertension in Cushing's syndrome, since considerable species differences exist with respect to the influence exerted by glucocorticoids on blood pressure.

In man, cortisol infusions for several days lead to an increase in cardiac output and in systolic blood pressure accompanied by sodium retention and an increase in body weight; plasma sodium concentration rises whereas plasma potassium as well as plasma renin concentration decrease. Plasma noradrenaline concentration has also been shown to fall after oral cortisol administration for several days. Therefore the renin–angiotensin system and the sympathetic nervous system probably do not play an important role in the development of glucocorticoid-induced hypertension. Glucocorticoid hormones cause a shift of sodium and fluid from the intra- to the extracellular compartment. The resulting increase in plasma volume probably contributes to the increase in cardiac output and thereby in systolic blood pressure. Various authors have regarded an increased vascular reactivity to adrenaline and noradrenaline as being important for the hypertensive effect of the glucocorticoids. In some studies, however, glucocorticoids were not found to exert any influence on vascular reactivity.

Mineralocorticoid excess syndromes (*primary aldosteronism, 11β-hydroxylase deficiency, 17α-hydroxylase deficiency*)

Mineralocorticoid-induced types of hypertension are *primary aldosteronism* due to an adrenocortical adenoma (Conn's syndrome) and hypertension caused by increased deoxycorticosterone formation due to congenital 11β-hydroxylase deficiency or congenital 17α-hydroxylase deficiency. In so-called *pseudo-primary aldosteronism* caused by a bilateral adrenal hyperplasia, the increased aldosterone formation is probably a concomitant phenomenon or a factor that intensifies, but does not actually cause, hypertension.

The precise mechanism of mineralocorticoid-induced hypertension has not as yet been clarified. It is well established, however, that the pressor effect of the mineralocorticoids is mediated by sodium chloride since the hypertensive effect was shown to be prevented by salt restriction. Exchangeable sodium and extracellular fluid volume are increased in patients with primary aldosteronism.

45

In normotensive subjects, oral administration of the synthetic mineralo-corticoid, fludrocortisone, leads to a blood-pressure increase resulting initially from a rise in the stroke volume and cardiac output. After a few weeks, the continuing increase in blood pressure is accompanied by a rise in total peripheral resistance, and cardiac output returns to normal. Patients with Conn's syndrome whose blood pressure has been normalized by admin-istration of the aldosterone antagonist, spironolactone, experience, after its discontinuation, a renewed rise in blood pressure. This results in the first few days from an increased cardiac output in the presence of a normal or even decreased total peripheral resistance. Eventually total peripheral resistance increases and cardiac output returns to normal. Thus, mineralocorticoid hypertension, like renal–parenchymatous hypertension, involves an inter-action between volume and vasoconstrictor factors, the latter ultimately prevailing. This evolution may be related to the concept of 'autoregulation' as referred to above.

Pheochromocytoma (See also Chapter 6)

Pheochromocytomas are tumours that derive from chromaffin cells of the adrenal medulla or the sympathetic trunk and lead to hypertension through increased catecholamine secretion. In rare cases, chromaffin tumours also develop from other neuroblastic or chemoreceptive cells. Less than 10% of the tumours are malignant pheochromoblastomas. Like normal medullo-adrenal tissue, pheochromocytomas contain dopamine, noradrenaline and adrenaline. The catecholamine content of pheochromocytomas is greatly increased compared with normal medulloadrenal tissue; the proportion of the individual catecholamines can vary widely.

Hypertension associated with pheochromocytoma is the only type of high blood pressure in which the aetiology has been clarified completely. The blood pressure elevation is due exclusively to an increase in circulating catecholamines. The increased catecholamine concentrations in plasma lead to a decrease in the number of adrenergic α and β receptors as well as to an impairment of receptor–effector coupling, the result being a reduced sensitivity to circulating and neurally released catecholamines.

The elevated catecholamine concentrations in plasma increase the contractility not only of the arterioles but also of the venous capacitance vessels, which leads to a reduction of plasma and blood volume. The hypovolaemia can result in orthostatic hypotension, the tendency towards the latter being promoted by the above-mentioned reduced sensitivity to neurally released noradrenaline. The hypertension usually disappears when the pheo-chromocytoma is removed (under the precautions indicated in Chapter 6).

HYPERTENSION ASSOCIATED WITH AORTIC COARCTATION

Hypertension associated with aortic coarctation is considered to be caused primarily by the flow obstacle in the isthmus area itself. In addition, an important role in the pathogenesis of hypertension associated with aortic coarctation was attributed to an adaptation of the baroreceptors to the pre-isthmical pressure elevations and to an increased renin secretion resulting from reduced renal perfusion.

DRUG-RELATED HYPERTENSION

Hypertension induced by oral contraceptives

The intake of oral contraceptives usually leads to a slight increase in blood pressure. About 5% of women who take contraceptives develop manifest hypertension; pre-existent hypertension can become worse. The risk of developing hypertension under the intake of contraceptives is increased in women with a familial history of hypertension, previous hypertension during pregnancy, overweight, diabetes mellitus or pre-existent nephropathy. The risk increases with age and is considerably greater in women over the age of 35 than in younger women. Both the oestrogen and progestagen components contribute to the development of hypertension.

The mechanism of the hypertensive effect of oral contraceptives has not yet been definitely clarified. The following concept was developed for a possible pathophysiological role of the renin–angiotensin system in the development of hypertension under contraceptives: oestrogens lead to an increased formation of angiotensin II and aldosterone; synthetic gestagens have a mineralocorticoid effect. The oestrogen-determined increase in aldosterone formation and the mineralocorticoid effect of the synthetic gestagens result in sodium retention, which leads to hypertension in predisposed women (see also Chapter 3).

Liquorice and indomethacin

Long-term intake of large amounts of liquorice can lead to the development of hypertension. The clinical symptoms resemble those of Conn's syndrome and the syndrome has therefore also been designated as 'pseudo-Conn's syndrome'. The symptoms are produced by glycoside derivatives of glycyrrhetinic acid contained in liquorice. Liquorice ingestion inhibits enzymes that inactivate both glucocorticoids and mineralocorticoids. The effect of this enzyme inhibition is an accumulation of glucocorticoid and mineralocorticoid hormones which are involved in the increased mineralocorticoid-like activity associated with liquorice ingestion. Blood-pressure elevations have also been observed in connection with the long-term application of indomethacin, which, among other things, inhibits the formation of vasodilatatory prostaglandins.

Selected references

Birkenhäger WH, de Leeuw PW (1979): Pathophysiological mechanisms in essential hypertension. *Pharmacol Ther* 8: 297.

Blaustein MP (1977): Sodium ions, calcium ions, blood pressure regulation and hypertension: a reassessment and a hypothesis. *Am J Physiol* 232: C165.

Brod J, Bahlmann J, Cachovan M, Pretschner P (1983): Development of hypertension in renal disease. *Clin Sci* 64: 141.

Curtis J, Luke R, Dustan H (1983): Remission of essential hypertension after renal transplantation. *N Engl J Med* 309: 1009.

De Wardener E, MacGregor GA (1982): The natriuretic hormone and essential hypertension. *Lancet* 1: 1450.

Esler M (1982): Assessment of sympathetic nervous function in humans from noradrenaline plasma kinetics. *Clin Sci* 62: 247.

Floras JS et al. (1988): Consequences of impaired arterial baroreflexes in essential hypertension: effects on pressor responses, plasma noradrenaline and blood pressure. *J Hypertension* 6: 525.

Folkow B (1982): Physiological aspects of primary hypertension. *Physiol Rev* 62: 348.

Folkow B (1971): The haemodynamic consequences of adaptive structural changes of the resistance vessels in hypertension. *Clin Sci* 41:1.

Goldstein DS (1981): Plasma noradrenaline in essential hypertension. *Hypertension* 3: 48.

Guyton AC (1981): Blood pressure regulation: Basic concepts. *Fed Proc* 40: 2252.

Hilton PJ (1986): Cellular sodium transport in essential hypertension. *N Engl J Med* 314: 222.

Julius S (1988): The blood pressure seeking properties of the central nervous system. *J Hypertension* 6: 177.

Luft FC, Weinberger MH, Grim CE (1982): Sodium sensitivity and resistance in normotensive humans. *Am J Med* 72: 726.

Lund-Johansen P (1983): Haemodynamics in essential hypertension – still an area of controversy. *J Hypertension* 1: 209.

Philipp Th, Distler A, Cordes U (1978): Sympathetic nervous system and blood pressure control in essential hypertension. *Lancet* ii: 959.

Postnov YV (1990): An approach to the explanation of cell membrane alteration in primary hypertension. *Hypertension* 15: 322.

Reaven GM (1988): Role of insulin resistance in human disease. *Diabetes* 37: 1595.

Rosendorf et al. (1985): Adrenergic receptors in hypertension. *Hypertension* 3: 571.

Strauer BE (1979): Ventricular function and coronary hemodynamics in hypertensive heart disease. *Am J Cardiol* 44: 999.

Tarazi RC et al. (1983): Can the heart initiate some forms of hypertension? *Fed Proc* 42: 2691.

Whitworth JA (1987): Mechanisms of glucocorticoid-induced hypertension. *Kidney Int* 31: 1213.

CHAPTER 3

Cardiovascular risk associated with hypertension; interactions with other risk indicators

JAN STAESSEN, ROBERT FAGARD and ANTOON AMERY

THE ASSOCIATION BETWEEN A RISK INDICATOR AND A DISEASE

A risk indicator is generally defined as a factor associated with the occurrence of a particular disease. The association between a risk factor and a disease is often, although not necessarily, causal. Risk is usually expressed as the relative increase or decrease in the probability of having or acquiring the disease when the risk indicator moves from one level to another. Risk estimates include random biological variation in the strength of the association between a particular risk factor and an illness. Thus, when a patient is a carrier of a certain risk factor, this does not automatically imply that he or she will become diseased.

A causal relationship is difficult to prove in observational epidemiological studies, but may be suspected when the association is significant and consistent through several populations; when the suspected causal factor precedes the occurrence of the disease; and when a plausible biological mechanism is available to explain the causal nature of the relationship. If a dose–response relationship between a risk factor and the incidence of a disease can be established, the likelihood of a causal association increases. Nonetheless, only intervention studies can prove the involvement of a risk factor in causing a disease. If modification of the risk factor consistently results in the anticipated change in disease incidence, then the causal nature of the association between risk indicator and disease may be considered to be scientifically proven.

THE ASSOCIATION BETWEEN BLOOD PRESSURE AND CARDIOVASCULAR RISK

Already by the mid-1960s the experience of life insurance companies indicated that even slight elevations above average of either systolic or diastolic blood pressure are associated with an increased mortality in younger and middle-aged subjects. Prospective epidemiological studies, such as the Framingham Study, have almost unanimously found a strongly positive association between blood pressure and the incidence of cardiovascular complications (Fig. 1).

THE MAIN POTENTIAL RISK FACTORS FOR ATHEROSCLEROSIS

* Age/male gender
* Hypertension
* Dyslipidaemia
* Truncal obesity
* Hyperuricaemia?
* Smoking
* Alcohol (via hypertension)
* Oral contraceptives
* Menopause

Elevation of blood pressure precedes the incidence of cardiovascular complications. Intervention studies have shown that the risk conferred by an elevated blood pressure is reversible by drug treatment. According to the results of a meta-analysis of 14 major prospective therapeutic trials, a fall in diastolic blood pressure of 5–6 mmHg was associated with an average reduction in the stroke rate of 42 (95% confidence interval 33–50%) and with a 14% reduction in the incidence of coronary heart disease (95% confidence interval 4–22%). Thus, the role of blood pressure elevation as a causal factor in the determination of cardiovascular risk has been established beyond any doubt, at least up to the age of 80 years.

In younger and middle-aged subjects, both systolic and diastolic blood pressure are related to cardiovascular risk. In older subjects, the incidence of cardiovascular complications is merely related to systolic pressure, diastolic blood pressure losing its predictive role. This predominance of systolic over diastolic pressure as a cardiovascular risk indicator in older people is not due to the larger range of systolic as compared with diastolic pressures, since this observation still holds, when systolic and diastolic blood are expressed on a similar scale in units of standard deviation (see also Chapter 5).

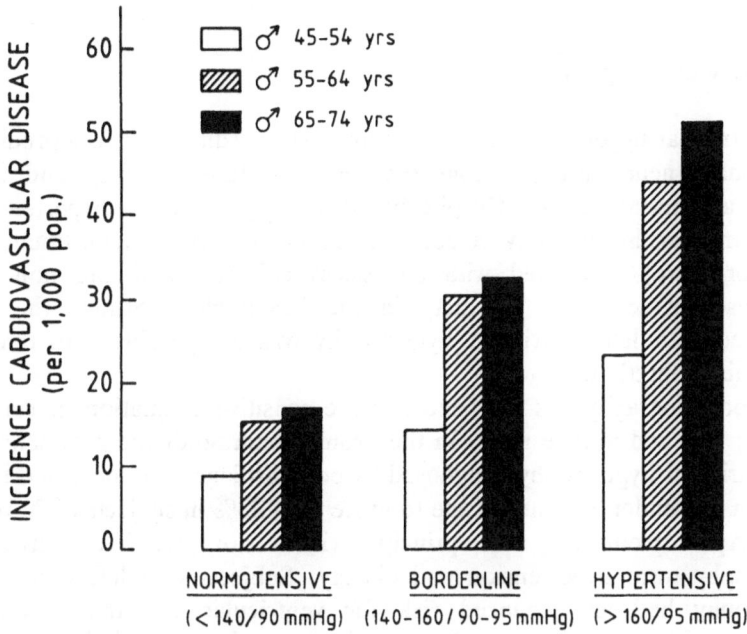

Fig. 1 20 years follow-up in Framingham Study (derived from results reported by the Framingham Group in *Bull NY Acad Med* (1988) 54: 573

INTERACTION OF HYPERTENSION WITH OTHER RISK INDICATORS

Age and gender

One of the misconceptions about hypertension is the idea that the increase in blood pressure with advancing age is a normal phenomenon compensating for the obstruction of blood flow in the hardened and stenotic arteries of elderly subjects. Another piece of conventional wisdom used to be that women tolerate hypertension better than men.

There is no evidence to support either of the above. On the contrary, while pressure does indeed rise with age, an examination of cardiovascular mortality and morbidity according to age shows no evidence whatsoever that hypertension is better tolerated in the old than in the young. As to the sex difference, it should be stressed that although the incidence of cardiovascular morbidity and mortality is greater in men than in women at any age and blood pressure level, the gradients of risk according to the blood pressure level are similar in both sexes.

Left ventricular hypertrophy

Left ventricular hypertrophy, diagnosed by electrocardiography, is a predictor of coronary heart disease, congestive heart failure, stroke, and even peripheral arterial disease. Despite being strongly related to hypertension, left ventricular hypertrophy remains independently (after adjustment for blood pressure) associated with an excess risk for fatal and non-fatal cardiovascular accidents. In fact, in the Framingham Study, the risk associated with left ventricular hypertrophy was comparable with that of myocardial infarction!

Echocardiography has provided a more sensitive estimation of cardiac chamber size and muscle mass. In the Framingham Study the prevalence of left ventricular hypertrophy, diagnosed by echocardiography, increased from less than 8% under 30 years of age to more than 33% in subjects of 70 years over. Apart from age, the principal risk factors for left ventricular hypertrophy were hypertension and obesity. Subjects with left ventricular hypertrophy had an enhanced risk for ventricular arrhythmias during ambulatory recordings of the electrocardiogram. In other clinical settings these ventricular arrhythmias were shown to predict sudden death. Thus it is obvious that left ventricular hypertrophy is associated with an increased risk for cardiovascular morbidity and mortality.

Hyperlipidaemia

In Western countries, many complications of hypertension, such as angina, myocardial infarction, atherothrombotic brain infarction, and claudication, are indirect ones in the sense that they are a consequence of the accelerated atherosclerosis in hypertensive patients. Hyperlipidaemia, particularly an elevated low-density lipoprotein cholesterol and a depressed high-density lipoprotein cholesterol, play an important role in the pathogenesis of atherosclerosis. Some investigators have even suggested that dyslipidaemia is a necessary prerequisite without which blood pressure elevation seldom leads to atherosclerotic complications.

Hyperlipidaemia and hypertension often occur in the same patient, and both conditions are independently associated with an increased sodium–lithium countertransport in the red cell membrane. The associations between hypertension and abnormal ion fluxes through the cell membranes are probably genetically determined, while raised plasma lipids and an increased sodium–lithium countertransport may both be the emanation of abnormalities in cell lipid metabolism. Whatever the underlying mechanism, when hyperlipidaemia and hypertension are diagnosed in the same patient, both conditions require treatment to prevent cardiovascular complications.

The intervention trials in hypertension have shown a reduction in the overall cardiovascular event rate and in stroke incidence by approximately 40%. However, the 14% reduction in the incidence of coronary heart disease observed in these intervention trials fell short of the 20–25% decrease that was expected from observational epidemiological studies. Coronary atherosclerosis is a chronic disease with multifactorial causation. Thus, blood pressure reduction over the relatively short time span in most intervention studies might just have been insufficient to completely normalise the excess risk of coronary accidents. As an additional explanation, it has been mentioned that diuretics were prescribed as a first-line hypotensive agent in nearly all intervention trials. It has been reported that diuretics raise the levels of both total and low-density cholesterol, but these reports involved only a small number of selected patients, followed for a maximum of a few months. Long-term allocation to hypotensive therapy with diuretics in the controlled randomized trials in hypertension demonstrated either no change, or only a marginal 1% rise in serum total cholesterol. Extrapolation from the cholesterol-lowering trials suggests that a 1% rise in serum total cholesterol would increase the incidence of coronary heart disease over a 5-year period by not more than 2%. Thus, small lipid differences associated with hypotensive treatment with diuretics or other hypotensive agents are very unlikely to account for more than a small fraction of the shortfall in the reduction of coronary events by hypotensive treatment.

Obesity

In adults living in countries with a Western lifestyle, a strong positive relationship between obesity and blood pressure has been demonstrated in cross-sectional and prospective epidemiological studies. In children and adolescents blood pressure rises very steeply with age for reasons which are not yet completely understood. In the young all indices of adiposity, such as absolute or relative body weight, the Quetelet or body mass index (kg/m^2), and skinfold thickness, are very closely correlated with blood pressure. After correction for body mass index, the relationship between chronological age and blood pressure in children and adolescents even disappears. Tracking for blood pressure and body weight can be easily demonstrated and the age-related increase in pressure in children and adolescents is proportional to the gain in body weight, childhood adiposity predisposing to hypertension during adult life (see also Chapter 5).

A positive relationship between blood pressure and adiposity is also present in most primitive societies. The observation that a relationship between body weight and blood pressure can be found in Western as well as in primitive societies is an argument in favour of the concept that the latter relationship is not due to confounding environmental factors, such as the intake of sodium, potassium, or alcohol, level of habitual physical activity, or social and psychological influences.

The issue of whether obesity, by itself, contributes to the risk of coronary heart disease has long been debated, since often obesity is accompanied by other coronary risk factors, such as hypertension, diabetes mellitus and hyperlipidaemia. However, several studies indicate that, when the multiple confounding factors are taken into account, obesity remains an independent risk factor for premature mortality.

Most studies have only considered body weight or body mass index, thereby diluting the importance of upper-body obesity as an important indicator of risk. In fact, coronary heart disease has been demonstrated to occur frequently in subjects with truncal obesity, with a waist to hip girth ratio >0.85. The association between upper body obesity, glucose intolerance, hypertriglyceridaemia and hypertension has been described as 'the deadly quartet' in view of the excess mortality associated with the condition. Insulin resistance and hyperinsulinaemia may be the key intermediary, explaining the relationship between these four and other factors.

THE MULTIFACTORIAL RISK COMPLEX

* Hypertension
* Tachycardia
* Truncal obesity   common cause
* Dyslipidaemia
* Glucose intolerance

Genetic clustering?
Insulin resistance/
hyperinsulinaemia?

Diabetes mellitus

Overt diabetes mellitus is a well-documented risk factor for coronary heart disease and cardiovascular and total mortality. While it is true that this risk is mediated in part by the association of diabetes with hypertension and other risk factors, it is generally accepted that overt or latent diabetes is a risk factor in its own right.

Hyperuricaemia

The association between hypertension and hyperuricaemia is well established. In normotensive subjects and in hypertensive patients, serum uric acid is inversely correlated with renal blood flow. It has been suggested that hyperuricaemia in hypertensive patients reflects the early stages of renal vascular involvement and nephrosclerosis.

Several investigators have studied the association between serum uric acid and cardiovascular morbidity, in particular coronary heart disease. On balance, most evidence fails to suggest that hyperuricaemia is independently related to the incidence of cardiovascular and coronary events.

Smoking

In the population there is aggregation between hypertension, smoking and alcohol intake. Smoking is an independent risk indicator for both myocardial infarction and stroke. The risk of experiencing a major coronary event, for pipe and cigar smokers is intermediate between the risks for non-smokers and cigarette smokers.

Although hypertension, smoking and hypercholesterolaemia confer approximately the same average increase in the risk of coronary heart disease, smoking in the presence of other risk factors, such as hypertension, has a synergistic effect on the morbidity and mortality from coronary events. Cessation of smoking results in a decreased mortality from coronary heart disease. The degree of risk reduction is dependent on the length of the time elapsed since cessation, the amount smoked, and the duration of smoking before cessation. Although the risk of coronary heart disease attributable to smoking is approximately halved one year after smoking cessation, it may take one decade before it approaches that of habitual non-smokers (see also Chapter 7).

Alcohol intake

The existence of a positive relationship between the use of alcohol and hypertension has been established by many cross-sectional and prospective epidemiological studies. There remains some difference of opinion on the questions of whether the relationship is linear or non-linear, and of whether blood pressure rises only beyond a certain threshold consumption of alcohol. On balance, most evidence suggests that the link between alcohol intake and the prevalence of hypertension can be uniformly demonstrated at a level of alcohol intake exceeding 3–5 drinks per day, whilst 1 or 2 drinks per day probably has no important effect on blood pressure.

Estimates of the proportion of alcohol-attributable hypertension in the population have ranged from 5 to 25% of all cases of blood pressure. Thus, assuming a causal relationship between alcohol intake and hypertension, it is possible that an excessive alcohol consumption represents the most common cause of secondary hypertension. As a consequence, a reduction of alcohol intake may well be an important preventive measure, and if the alcohol-related hypertension is reversible, also a therapeutic step in the management of hypertension (see Chapter 7).

Use of contraceptive pills

Women taking combined oestrogen–progestagen pills show a small increase in blood pressure, averaging 3–5 mmHg for systolic and 1–2 mmHg for diastolic pressure. However, in some women, the rise in pressure is marked, and in a few severe hypertension may develop. Thus, contraceptive pill use causes a 3- to 6-fold rise in the risk of overt hypertension. The risk of hypertension attributable to oral contraceptives in women has been reported to increase with age, becoming substantial only in women over 35 years or older. The risk also rises proportionally with the duration of contraceptive pill intake. It seems plausible that factors, such as a positive family history of hypertension or a history of renal disease may also increase the risk of hypertension, attributable to the use of birth control pills, but this has not yet been proven.

Oral contraceptives decrease glucose tolerance in most women. The effect averages approximately 10 mg/dl one hour after a glucose load and is unrelated to the duration of oral contraceptive use but is additive to the effects of age, obesity, and a family history of diabetes, all of which decrease glucose tolerance.

All progestagens, currently used in oral contraceptives produce a decrease in high-density lipoprotein (HDL) cholesterol, mainly in HDL_2-cholesterol which is believed to be the cardioprotective subfraction of HDL-cholesterol. The degree of the decrease in HDL-cholesterol is related to the amount and the potency of the progestagen. Because the oestrogen component of birth control pills produces alterations in the HDL-cholesterol levels in the opposite direction, the net effect of any oral contraceptive formulation on HDL-cholesterol depends entirely on its composition.

The effects of birth control pills on blood pressure, glucose tolerance and HDL-cholesterol have raised the suspicion that oral contraceptives may augment the risk of arterial thrombosis and possibly accelerate athero-sclerosis. Older epidemiological studies at first confirmed this suspicion and demonstrated that women on the contraceptive pill, in comparison with controls of similar age, had a higher incidence of myocardial infarction and stroke, especially if they were older than 35 years of age. More recent studies suggest however that the use of contraceptive formulations containing less than 50 μg oestrogen by healthy non-smoking women up to the age of 45 is not associated with an increased incidence of cardiovascular disease. However, oral contraceptives should not be prescribed to women with hyper-tension or any pre-existing systemic disease that may affect the cardiovascular system, nor to women over 35 years who smoke.

Menopause

Postmenopausal subjects and women who have undergone bilateral ovarectomy have a higher risk of coronary heart disease than premenopausal women of similar age. Postmenopausal women are more prone to develop atherosclerosis since they tend to have higher blood levels of triglycerides, and (very low- and low-density lipoprotein) cholesterol. Whether blood pressure increases following menopause and thereby contributes to the enhanced cardiovascular risk profile of postmenopausal women remains debatable.

Selected references

Amery A, Fagard R, Staessen J (1987): Recent data on changes in lipid metabolism induced by hypotensive drugs. *Curr Opinion Cardiol* 2: 769–774.

Carr SJ, Thomas TH, Laker MF, Wilkinson R (1990): Elevated sodium–lithium countertransport: a familial marker of hyperlipidaemia and hypertension. *J Hypertension* 8: 139–146.

Collins R, Peto R, MacMahon S, Hebert P, Fiebach NH, Eberlein KA, Godwin J, Qizilbash N, Taylor JO, Hennekens CH (1990): Blood pressure, stroke, and coronary heart disease. Part 2, short-term reductions in blood pressure: overview of randomised drug trials in their epidemiological context. *Lancet* 1: 827–838.

Fielding JE (1985): Smoking: health effects and control. *N Engl J Med* 313: 491–498.

Handbook of Hypertension (Series Editors WH Birkenhäger, JL Reid). Volume 12. Hypertension in the Elderly (Eds. A Amery, J Staessen). Elsevier, Amsterdam, 1989.

Handbook of Hypertension (Series Editors WH Birkenhäger, JL Reid). Volume 6. Epidemiology of Hypertension. (Ed. CJ Bulpitt). Elsevier, Amsterdam, 1985.

Kannel WB (1974): Role of blood pressure in cardiovascular epidemiology. *Prog Cardiovasc Dis* 17: 5–24.

Kannel WB (1976): Some lessons in cardiovascular epidemiology from Framingham. *Am J Cardiol* 37: 269–282.

Kannel WB (1990): Contribution of the Framingham Study to preventive cardiology. *J Am Coll Cardiol* 15: 206–211.

Kaplan NM (1989): The deadly quartet. Upper-body obesity, glucose intolerance, hypertriglyeridaemia, and hypertension. *Arch Intern Med* 149: 1514–1520.

Klatsky AL, Friedman GD, Siegelaub AB (1981): Alcohol use and cardiovascular disease: the Kaiser-Permanente experience. *Circulation* 64 (Suppl III): III32–III41.

Levy D (1988): Left ventricular hypertrophy. Epidemiological insights from the Framingham Heart Study. *Drugs* Suppl 5: 1–5.

Levy D, Garrison RJ, Savage DD, Kannel WB, Castelli WP (1990): Prognostic implications of echocardiographically determined left ventricular mass in the Framingham Heart Study. *N Engl J Med* 322: 1561–1566.

MacMahon SW, Peto R, Cutler J, Collins R, Sorlie P, Neaton J, Abbott R, Godwin J, Dyer A, Stamler J (1990): Blood pressure, stroke, and coronary heart disease. Part 1, prolonged differences in blood pressure: prospective observational studies corrected for the regression dilution bias. *Lancet* 335: 765–774.

Stadel BV (1981): Oral contraceptives and cardiovascular disease. *N Engl J Med* 305: 672–677.

Staessen J, Fagard R, Van Hoof R, Amery A (1988): Mortality in various intervention trials in elderly hypertensive patients. *Eur Heart J* 9: 215–222.

Staessen J, Fagard R, Amery A (1988): The relationship between body weight and blood pressure. *J Human Hypertension* 2: 207–217.

Staessen J, Bulpitt CJ, Fagard R, Lijnen P, Amery P (1989): The influence of menopause on blood pressure. *J Human Hypertension* 3: 427–433.

Stampfer MJ, Willett WC, Colditz GA, Speizer FE, Hennekens CH (1988): Prospective study of past use of oral contraceptive agents and risk of cardiovascular diseases. *N Engl J Med* 319: 1313–1317.

CHAPTER 4

Evaluation of the hypertensive subject

LENNART HANSSON and ANDERS SVENSSON

INTRODUCTION

When evaluating an individual with newly detected elevated blood pressure a few rather simple rules can be followed. One of those rules is to obtain the maximal amount of information about the patient at the lowest possible cost. In other words, in all diagnostic work-up the cost–benefit ratio should be as high as possible.

A second important consideration is that no diagnostic work-up should be performed if the results are not going to be employed in the clinical care or treatment of the patient. In other words, diagnostic work-up for purely academic reasons should be avoided.

With these two simple rules in mind, the purpose of this chapter is to discuss (1) evaluation of the middle-of-the-road hypertensive, (2) screening for curable hypertensive states, and (3) assessment of other risk factors and target organ damage.

EVALUATION OF THE MIDDLE-OF-THE-ROAD HYPERTENSIVE

A few decades ago widely diverging views were expressed regarding the amount and extent of work-up that was called for in hypertension. On the one extreme, it was argued that a complete work-up was mandatory for every hypertensive patient, meaning that all forms of secondary hypertension should be excluded with the greatest degree of certainty. This meant extensive laboratory testing and X-ray investigations in every patient with hypertension.

The other extreme view was that since the yield of diagnostic work-up in terms of finding secondary forms of hypertension was minimal, all diagnostic work-up could be neglected. Instead antihypertensive treatment with the cheapest available drugs should be instituted. This way, it was claimed, benefit would be maximal and costs minimal.

As usual, the truth of the matter probably lies somewhere in between the extremes. On the following pages a diagnostic work-up suitable for the middle-of-the-road hypertensive patient will be described. There are at least four important reasons for making an initial work-up in all patients with newly detected hypertension. These are:

AIMS OF INITIAL WORK-UP IN HYPERTENSIVES

* To find hypertensives with secondary forms of hypertension, which may be curable (see below).

* To find hypertensives with particularly poor prognosis (left ventricular hypertrophy, renal impairment, etc.).

* To find hypertensives with additional risk factors for cardiovascular disease, e.g. cigarette smoking, lipid abnormalities, disturbed glucose metabolism, etc.

* To find factors of importance for the choice of antihypertensive therapy.

The extent of diagnostic work-up

All diagnostic work-up probably benefits from a more-or-less rigidly structured scheme meaning that all individuals go through a standardized procedure.

In brief, the three main components of the diagnostic work-up for hypertension is very similar to that of any other diagnostic work-up. It consists of a careful history, a physical examination and evaluation of relevant laboratory tests.

History

A correct history is an invaluable corner-stone of any diagnostic work-up. For hypertension the following items are of particular value:

Family history

The subject should be questioned about hypertension, cardiovascular mortality at young age, diabetes and renal disease in the family. The purpose here is to identify patients who may have a poor prognosis.

Social factors

Questions about profession, experience of stress at home or at work, family relations etc. may yield significant clues. Interest in factors such as these seem to be increasing, although it is difficult at the present time to fully evaluate their influence with regard to hypertension and cardiovascular disease.

Dietary and hygienic factors

Smoking habits, alcohol intake, excessive sodium consumption etc. should be recorded.

Previous morbidity

Emphasis here should be on the history of previous cardiovascular disorders (angina pectoris, myocardial infarction, intermittent claudication, cerebro-vascular episodes, etc.) since such disorders would increase the risk for further cardiovascular morbidity.

In addition, possible symptoms from the kidneys and urinary tract should be recorded.

Symptoms of gout, chronic bronchitis or bronchial asthma may affect the choice of antihypertensive therapy and should therefore be recorded.

Gynecology and obstetrics

The number of pregnancies, possible problems during pregnancy (oedema, proteinuria, excessive increase in weight, hypertension, etc.) should be recorded. The use of birth control pills should be clarified.

Current symptoms

Questions about severe headaches, visual disturbances, nose bleedings, etc. should be asked. Such symptoms should lead to the suspicion of malignant hypertension which is almost invariably associated with symptoms.

There should also be questions about paroxysmal episodes of paleness and sweating, possibly together with headaches and palpitations, which should lead to the suspicion of pheochromocytoma. Muscle fatigue, vertigo and nocturia may be of interest and should lead to the suspicion of aldosteronism.

A number of other symptoms, e.g. from the kidneys or the urinary tract, may also indicate secondary forms of hypertension. It should be remembered that uncomplicated essential hypertension rarely gives symptoms.

Therapy

Ongoing medical therapy as well as previous treatment with antihypertensive drugs must be recorded. Possible previous side-effects should also be penetrated.

A brief history of this kind can be recorded in a short period of time. Needless to say, further in-depth penetration is needed on issues where the patient has given a positive reply.

Physical examination

A number of organ systems need to be examined in the physical examination. Most important of all the steps here is the measurement of blood pressure, which hasv been dealt with in Chapter 1.

Examination of the heart

The heart is examined in the standard fashion by using inspection, palpation and auscultation. An accentuated second tone over the aorta is a frequent finding in hypertension and carries no particular significance other than as a marker of the elevated arterial pressure.

It is more important to listen for third and fourth sounds which may indicate left ventricular failure. The physical findings should then be related to other examinations, in particular the electrocardiogram.

Lung examination

A standardized lung examination is performed aiming at identifying obstructive pulmonary disease or signs of left ventricular failure.

Vascular examinations

Palpation of pulses in various vascular beds should be performed. Most important is a reduced amplitude and/or delayed pulse in the femoral artery which may suggest coarctation of the aorta. The best way to establish this is to simultaneously palpate the radial and femoral pulse.

The carotid arteries should also be examined both by palpation and auscultation.

Finally one should listen for bruits over the renal arteries. This can be done from both the ventral and dorsal sides of the patient. From the ventral side it is done by pressing the diaphragm of the stethoscope rather firmly against the abdominal wall in order to compress underlying hollow organs. This will improve transmission of the rather weak sounds originating from turbulent flow, e.g. distal to a renal artery stenosis.

Eye-ground examination

In all patients with newly detected hypertension the eye-ground should be inspected (Fig. 1). This examination is mandatory in all patients with markedly elevated blood pressure, i.e. diastolic blood pressures ⩾ 120 mmHg and in patients with symptoms. The main objective is to diagnose and/or exclude malignant hypertension (Fig. 2).

Other examinations

A number of other organ systems need to be evaluated. In particular, possible neurological dificits and thyroid abnormalities should be considered.

Basal laboratory investigation

Certain basal laboratory investigations of blood and urine are important in the diagnostic work-up of patients with hypertension.

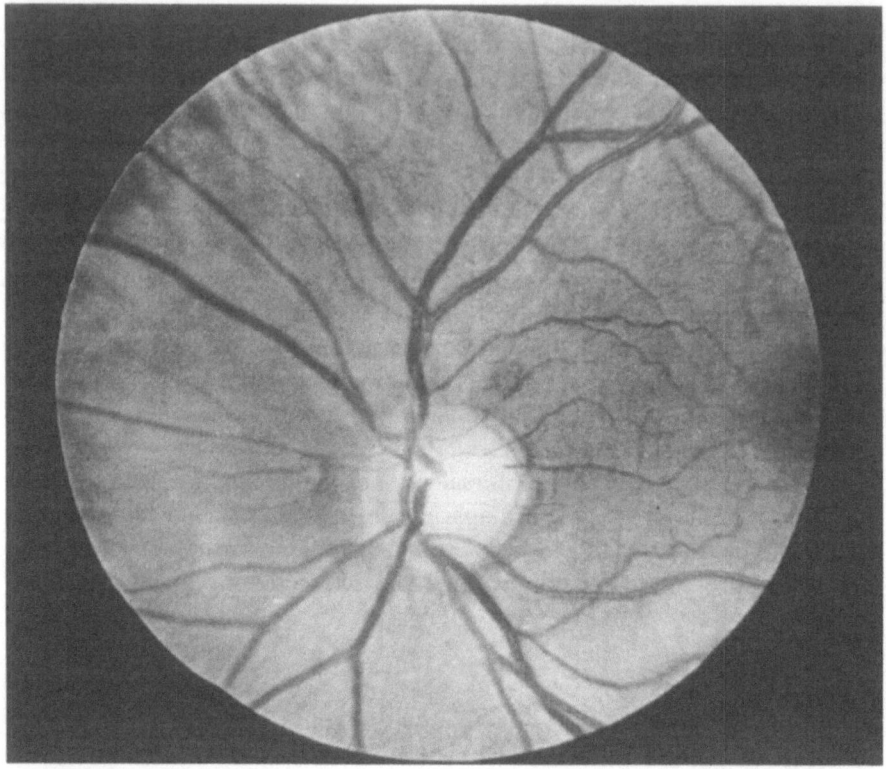

Fig. 1 A normal eye-ground showing approximately the same diameter of the veins (dark) and of the arteries, a sharply delineated papilla, no haemmorhages or exudates and no A–V nipping where arteries cross veins

Serum electrolytes

An evaluation of serum potassium and serum sodium should always be made. One should be aware of the fact that, in particular, serum potassium can be markedly affected by a faulty technique, i.e. prolonged stasis or muscle work when taking the blood sample and haemolysis in the test tube. All these circumstances will lead to an increased serum potassium level. Serum potassium is of great importance since a low value may indicate primary or secondary aldosteronism. By relating serum potassium to serum sodium a certain guidance to secondary or primary aldosteronism can be obtained.

Serum calcium is frequently analysed in the routine work-up of hypertensive patients. It is important to find patients with hyperparathyroidism, who frequently also have hypertension. A serum calcium in the upper range of normal should probably preclude the use of thiazide diuretics.

Any abnormalities with regard to serum electrolytes should lead to further history taking with regard to the use of diuretics or purgatives as well as regarding the consumption of liquorice. Before going ahead with an expanded diagnostic work-up the tests should always be repeated.

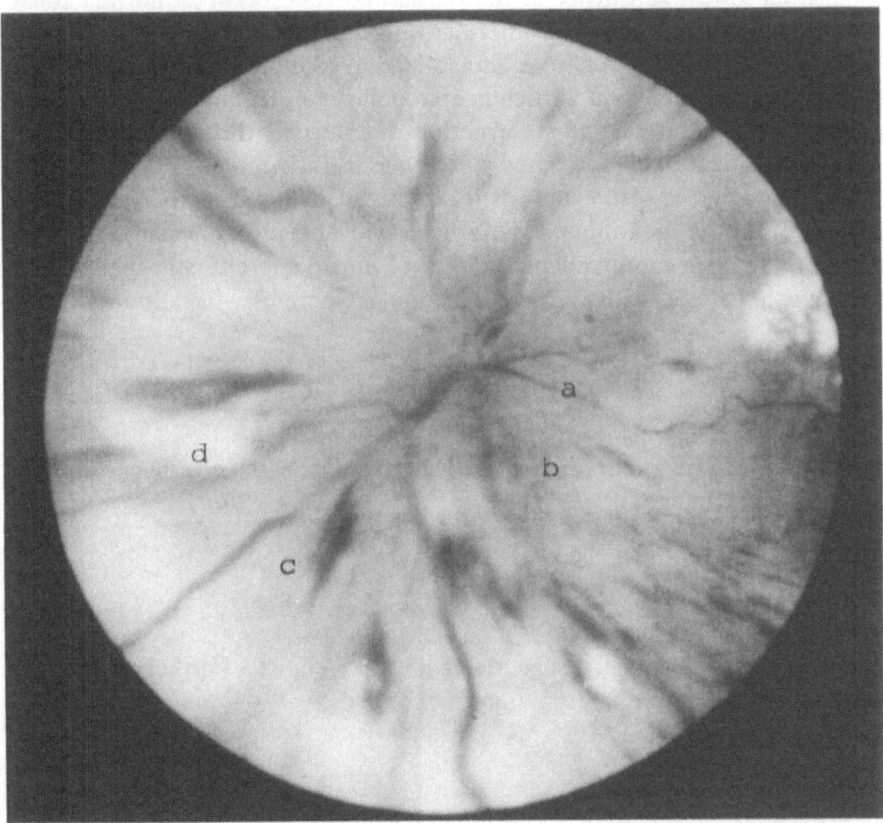

Fig 2. An eye-ground with degree IV changes (fundus hypertonicus IV) corresponding to malignant hypertension. The arterioles are markedly constricted (a) having a much smaller diameter than the veins. The papilla can not be clearly defined due to papilloedema (b) and there are numerous haemmorhages and exudates, e.g. c and d. These dramatic changes are comparatively easy to diagnose even for someone who is not a trained ophthalmologist and since they should initiate immediate action (hospitalization of the patient) it is important that this examination is not neglected, particularly in new patients presenting with marked elevation of blood pressure and usually one or more symptoms, e.g. headache, blurred vision, etc.

Serum creatinine

Determination of serum creatinine is probably the simplest and most important clinical examination of the patient's renal function. Thus, an elevated value may indicate primary renal disease or renal damage secondary to the elevated blood pressure. However, it should be borne in mind that this test has its lowest sensitivity in the borderline zone between normal renal function and slightly reduced glomerular filtration rate.

An elevated serum creatinine should lead to caution in the use of certain antihypertensive agents, in particular spironolactone. It should also be borne in mind that the diuretic and antihypertensive effects of thiazide diuretics are reduced in patients with decreased glomerular filtration rates.

In some centres serum urea is used instead of, or in parallel with, the analysis of serum creatinine. The greatest advantage of measuring serum urea is that it is a more reliable marker of impending uraemia than serum creatinine in patients with marked reduction in glomerular filtration rate.

Protein in urine

Proteinuria may be a marker of underlying renal disease or of hypertension-induced renal damage.

Glucose in urine

Glucose in urine strongly suggests diabetes mellitus. Further diagnostic work-up is required if glucose is found in the urine.

Blood glucose

In many centres blood glucose is becoming a routine test in the work-up of hypertensive patients. This is due to the growing awareness of the link between arterial hypertension and diabetes mellitus or pre-diabetic changes of glucose and insulin metabolism.

Electrocardiogram

A full electrocardiogram, including chest and extremity leads, should always be performed. This may give an indication of left ventricular hypertrophy, conduction disturbances, previous silent infarcts etc. The existence of A–V block II and III contraindicates the use of β-adrenoreceptor blocking agents and some calcium-blocking drugs.

Desirable but not mandatory tests

A number of other laboratory tests can be useful in the diagnostic work-up of hypertensive patients, although we are somewhat hesitant to list them as mandatory investigations in all patients. Of great value would be:

1. An echocardiographic examination of the heart. This is the best way of diagnosing left ventricular hypertrophy which in itself contributes to an increased risk of several cardiovascular complications.
2. A urine sediment examination was previously often performed in the diagnostic work-up of hypertension. The findings may be difficult to evaluate for an untrained examinor, but an adequately performed study can be of great help for the diagnosis of chronic renal disease, e.g. chronic pyelonephritis.
3. Serum urate is in itself a weak risk indicator. Slightly elevated levels are frequently seen in hypertensive patients and values in the high normal range should lead to caution in the use of thiazide diuretics.
4. Serum lipoproteins may constitute important additional risk indicators and are dealt with separately in a subsection of this chapter (see below).

Studies which are not mandatory

Chest X-ray

In most patients with uncomplicated hypertension a chest X-ray can be replaced by a careful physical heart–lung examination and an electro-cardiogram.

Intravenous pyelography

The i.v.p. is usually of even less importance than a chest X-ray in the diagnostic work-up of hypertensive patients. Only if there are special reasons, e.g. the suspicion of renal forms of hypertension, should this investigation be performed.

If an i.v.p. is performed as part of the diagnostic work-up in hypertension, particularly in the presence of suspected renal artery stenosis, it should be performed as a rapid sequence pyelogram. Positive findings, suggesting renal artery stenosis, should be confirmed or excluded by renal arteriography.

Radiorenography

Isotope renography can, at least in some specialized centres, be a very useful tool for diagnosis of, and particularly for the exclusion of, renal artery stenosis. In most hands, however, this method appears to have about the same specificity/sensitivity as the rapid sequence i.v.p. In other words, both these methods are not usually providing a screening method for renal artery stenosis of sufficiently high validity.

Digital angiography

This is probably the best screening method for renal artery stenosis short of renal arteriography.

Catecholamines in urine

There is no need for analysis of catecholamines in urine in the routine diagnostic work-up of hypertension. However, if there are signs or symptoms indicative of pheochromocytoma, this study should be performed, usually on three separate 24-hour urine collections. Analysis of metanephrines in urine probably offers a higher degree of sensitivity than that of standard catecholamines, which, in turn is better than that of vanillylmandelic acid (VMA).

Summary

A simple diagnostic work-up for the middle-of-the-road hypertensive patient along the lines suggested here should be sufficient to identify most of the secondary forms of hypertension, e.g. chronic renal disease, renovascular hypertension and coarctation of the aorta. It must be underlined, however, that none of these disorders will be diagnosed with full certainty by the procedures suggested here. However, in practical terms, this will probably be of little significance, since most forms of secondary hypertension will be treated with pharmacological agents anyway. The curable forms of secondary hypertension will be dealt with briefly below and in greater detail in Chapter 8.

Another advantage the diagnostic work-up outlined here is that additional risk factors for cardiovascular disease, e.g. smoking, lipid abnormalities etc., will be identified and adequate measures against these factors can be instituted as well. Finally, a simple diagnostic work-up of this kind will provide some background for the choice of suitable antihypertensive therapy.

SCREENING FOR CURABLE HYPERTENSION STATES (See also Chapter 8)

Most of the curable forms of hypertension should be diagnosed or suspected already from the initial work-up as outlined above. Further diagnostic investigation may be required to establish the exact nature of the secondary cause, however.

Coarctation of the aorta should be suspected based upon the pulse palpation or the measurement of blood pressure in the leg as described above.

A number of renal forms of hypertension, many of which are not curable, should be suspected by the careful taking of history and the assessment of laboratory findings. Of particular interest is renovascular hypertension, which may give rise to bruits over the renal arteries, electrolyte disturbances or an increase in serum creatinine. From a practical point of view, these patients also often have rather marked elevations of blood pressure and may be difficult to treat with common antihypertensive drugs. When this happens further investigation should be considered.

A number of endocrine forms of hypertension give rise to symptoms or laboratory abnormalities. Thus, patients with primary aldosteronism frequently have low serum potassium values. Sometimes these patients also complain of nocturia and muscle weakness, both of which are linked to the low serum potassium concentration.

Patients with pheochromocytoma may complain of attacks of headaches, paleness and sweating. Even more common is a finding of subfebrile temperature.

Cushing's syndrome and acromegaly should be suspected based on physical findings.

Hyperparathyroidism should be suspected based mainly on an elevated serum calcium concentration.

Finally, drug-induced hypertension, e.g. due to birth control pills, oestrogens, intake of abnormal levels of liquorice etc., should be picked up when taking the medical history.

Many of the curable secondary forms of hypertension require further investigation and such studies should usually be performed in specialized centres as their interpretation may require expertise.

EXAMINATION OF THE HYPERTENSIVE SUBJECT

History
    personal
        life events
        symptoms
        medication
    family
        hypertension, premature death

Physical examination
        blood pressure series
        pulse rate
        heart, lungs, kidneys
        arteries
        eye grounds

Laboratory
    urinalysis
    serum/blood
        creatinine/urea
        electrolytes
        glucose, lipids, uric acid
    electrocardiogram

        EXTEND EXAMINATION IF
        SUGGESTIVE FOR SECONDARY
        HYPERTENSION OR TARGET ORGAN
        DAMAGE

OTHER RISK FACTORS

Hypertension is one of the major risk factors for cardiovascular disease, the most common cause of death in the industrialized world. There are, however, several other factors that are associated with cardiovascular morbidity and mortality which themselves increase the risk. These other risk factors interact with hypertension and can amplify the negative effects of elevated blood pressure in the susceptible individual (see also Chapter 3)..

Some of the risk factors are amenable to intervention while others can only be noted but not influenced. However, they can help us to decide how best to take care of the individual patient, even if the risk factor as such cannot be reduced.

Some risk factors are linked to the individual, such as sex, age, race and hereditary influence and can only be noted, Others are related to life style, e.g. smoking, the use of alcohol, physical activity and the use of contraceptive pills. Others still are biochemical risk factors, for example glucose intolerance, hypercholesterolaemia, proteinuria and increased levels of plasma fibrinogen.

Some risk factors can be identified in the patient by making a routine physical examination (obesity, waist/hip ratio, tachycardia) and most of the others by direct questioning (e.g. smoking, heredity, perhaps alcohol, physical activity, social class and shift work).

Age is of great importance in this context. Blood pressure in most populations increases until about 60 years of age. Independently of blood pressure, the risk of having a myocardial infarction or a stroke increases with age, but, when hypertension is added, the risk of having a cardiocerebro-vascular complication is even higher.

Obviously, nothing can be done about age or gender. It is well known that women before menopause have a lower risk of having cardiovascular complications than men. In the Framingham study, 45–74-year-old males had about twice the incidence of cardiovascular death during 20 years of follow-up as compared with women of equal age. This holds true for normotensive as well as hypertensive individuals, but it is important to remember that, for both men and women, the risk of cardiovascular death is tripled in hypertension compared with normotension.

Heredity seems to be of importance, and, according to some studies, hypertension as well as complications such as stroke, are more related to high maternal blood pressure and cerebrovascular disease. This could be interpreted to mean that purely genetic factors are not solely responsible. Most children spend more time with their mother than their father, and diet, for example, is more influenced by the mother. Perhaps intrauterine environmental factors are of importance since retarded intrauterine growth has been found to be associated with haemodynamic changes in the fetus, with increased peripheral vascular resistance being observed. Whether this is of importance for the early development of the cardiovascular system is not known, but children born small for gestational age have higher blood pressure than those born normal for gestational age, and this difference remains in young adults.

Body weight is related to blood pressure. Hypertensive patients have, on the average, higher body weight than the population in general. Weight is an independent risk factor for cardiovascular disease that can be influenced. Weight reduction in overweight subjects also has a direct effect on the blood pressure and is therefore an important non-pharmacological measure.

The location of the excess fat is also important. Waist/hip ratio, i.e. the ratio between waist and hip circumference, is independently associated with cardiovascular disease. The female type with wide hips is less ominous than the male type of overweight with a big belly and increased waist/hip ratio.

Diabetes in combination with hypertension has a poor prognosis. Both hypertension and diabetes accelerate the atherosclerotic process, and when combined the result is often serious complications, such as stroke or myocardial infarction, at a relatively young age. Rapid decline of kidney function is another hallmark of the hypertensive diabetic patient.

Proteinuria is another risk factor, but is also a sign of renal damage that might be an effect of elevated blood pressure. The same could be said for left ventricular hypertrophy, which is a sign of target organ damage as well as an indicator of a less favourable prognosis.

When it comes to risk factors, the two most important in this context are smoking and hypercholesterolaemia. The reason for this is two-fold. Firstly, they are strongly related to cardiovascular disease and mortality, and secondly, and most important, they can be reduced.

The object of treating hypertensive patients is to reduce, and if possible, normalize, the increased cardiovascular mortality and morbidity. To achieve maximal effect, reduction of blood pressure is not always enough. Other risk factors should also be considered, and it is as important to get smokers with hypertension to quit smoking as it is to normalize their blood pressure. However, it is often more difficult to achieve success in getting smokers to quit than to successfully treat hypertension. In this common situation, it is even more important to reduce those risk factor(s) that can be influenced. Normalization of blood pressure thus is more important in a smoking patient.

Hypercholesterolaemia is another strong risk factor for cardiovascular disease together with hypertension and smoking the most important. It is therefore applicable to use the same line of reasoning as with smoking: if cholesterol cannot be normalized, it is even more important to achieve adequate blood pressure control.

72

In the evaluation of the hypertensive patient, other risk factors for cardiovascular disease should be considered. The factors that can be changed to reduce the risk, without harm to the patient, should of course be influenced. The risk factors that can only be observed and identified but not influenced are nevertheless of importance. They can help us pick out the individuals who will benefit most from antihypertensive treatment, since hypertension and other risk factors are additive or act synergistically to cause cardiovascular disease and premature death.

TARGET ORGAN DAMAGE

Long-standing hypertension will sooner or later result in organ damage. Part of this process will be accelerated in patients with other risk factors, but in general, hypertensive organ damage develops gradually over years and maybe decades.

One very important exception is the arteriolar necrosis that is the hallmark of malignant hypertension. In this condition, vascular damage develops very rapidly once the malignant phase has begun. In the retinal vessels, the result of fibrinoid arteriolar necrosis will be haemorrhages and 'cotton-wool' spots, findings that define the condition known as malignant hypertension (Fig. 2). In the kidneys, the rapid deterioration of renal function is characteristic of malignant hypertension, and renal failure has been the major cause of death. However, with adequate therapy the retinal changes are rapidly reversible, and renal function may improve, or at least not deteriorate further, if not too far advanced before treatment is started.

Non-malignant hypertension causes other types of vascular damage. It should perhaps be pointed out that, with the possible exception of hypertensive heart disease, practically all clinical manifestations of hypertension are related to vascular damage.

There are two distinctive forms of arterial disease in hypertension. The hypertrophy of the smooth muscle layer of the vessel walls of the small arteries and arterioles are directly related to the height of the blood pressure, and can be reduced or prevented, at least partly, by adequate blood pressure reduction. On the other hand, hypertension is but one of several major risk factors for the development of atherosclerotic lesions in large arteries. These lesions are often present in normotensive individuals and antihypertensive treatment has been less successful in reducing this kind of vascular disease.

In the small vessels, hypertrophy of the smooth muscle layer is not the only consequence of hypertension. Perhaps the most pronounced changes occur within the intima, which normally consists of only one or two layers of cells. In hypertension, cellular proliferation of the intima is characteristic.

There is also often proliferation of the elastic layers and sometimes deposition of amorphous material, known as hyalinization. The result is reduced vascular lumen, increased resistance and reduced blood flow. In organs like skeletal muscle and the skin, the main consequence of this change of vessel design is increased vascular resistance that serves to further increase blood pressure. Here the possible reduction of blood flow will have relatively minor consequences.

In long-standing severe hypertension, decreased renal function due to hypertensive changes known as nephrosclerosis has not been uncommon. Proteinuria and reduced glomerular filtration due to this condition are rare today, now that most hypertensive patients are treated with effective antihypertensive drugs. Another cause of reduced renal function in hypertension is the development of atherosclerotic renal artery stenosis with reduced blood flow to the kidney on the affected side. Noticeable reductions of kidney function due to this cause will be seen with bilateral stenoses or when the contralateral kidney has a previously reduced function.

Non-haemorrhagic brain infarction is by far the most common form of stroke and is strongly correlated to hypertension. The risk of having a non-haemorrhagic stroke has been calculated to be increased by a factor of 8–10 in hypertensive individuals, while the risk for haemorrhagic stroke is three times that in normotensives,

Hypertensive heart disease was previously a common cause of congestive heart failure and death. With effective treatment, overt hypertensive heart failure due to high afterload (i.e. very high blood pressure due to elevated peripheral resistance) has become rare. Unfortunately coronary heart disease thus far has proven to be rather resistant in the face of antihypertensive treatment.

The heart will respond with hypertrophy to the increase of its workload in hypertension. Left ventricular hypertrophy occurs very rapidly in experimental hypertension, since cellular protein synthesis increases within hours when blood pressure is raised. In young patients and children with mildly elevated blood pressure or borderline hypertension, echocardiographic signs of left ventricular hypertrophy can be detected. These early structural cardiac changes may be partly genetically determined.

Left ventricular hypertrophy is a consequence of hypertension and is also an important risk factor for cardiovascular disease, including angina pectoris, myocardial infarction, arrhythmias, stroke, intermittent claudication and congestive heart failure. Older studies used electrocardiography (ECG) to identify left ventricular hypertrophy. In recent years, echocardiography has been used as a much more sensitive method to diagnose hypertrophy of the heart. It has been clearly demonstrated that even the less pronounced changes that can be detected by echocardiography are associated with an increased risk for cardiovascular disease and mortality.

Selected references

1988 Joint National Committee: The 1988 report of the Joint National Committee on detection, evaluation and treatment of high blood pressure. *Arch Intern Med* 148: 1023–1028.

Kannel WB, Stokes J III (1985): Hypertension as a cardiovascular risk factor. In Handbook of Hypertension (Series Editors WH Birkenhäger, JL Reid), Volume 6: Epidemiology of Hypertension (Ed. CJ Bulpitt). Elsevier Science Publishers BV, Amsterdam pp. 15–34.

Levy D (1988): Left ventricular hypertrophy. Epidemiological insights from the Framingham Heart Study. *Drugs* Suppl 5: 1–5.

Menard J, Degoulet P, Chatellier G, Corvol P (1983): The assessment, investigation and care of the hypertensive patient. In Handbook of Hypertension (Series Editors WH Birkenhager, JL Reid), Volume 1: Clinical Aspects of Essential Hypertension (Ed. JIS Robertson). Elsevier Science Publishers BV, Amsterdam, pp. 493–502.

Schmieder RE, Messerli FH, Sturgill D *et al.* (1989): Cardiac performance after reduction of myocardial hypertrophy. *Am J Med* 87: 22–27.

WHO/ISH Fifth Mild Hypertension Conference: 1989 Guidelines for the Management of Mild Hypertension: Memorandum from a WHO/ISH meeting. *J Hypertension* 7: 689–693.

CHAPTER 5

Special situations in hypertension (childhood and adolescence; pregnancy; old age)

LAWRENCE J. BEILIN

CHILDREN AND ADOLESCENTS

Blood pressure measurement (see also Chapter 1)

In infants, blood pressures are best recorded either using a mercury column and cuff with a Doppler ultrasound device to detect pulsation, or by oscillometric techniques. In older children and adolescents standard sphygmomanometry is still the cheapest and most reliable method for clinical practice, but cuff size is criticial. Too small a cuff will over-estimate pressures. If possible a cuff in which the inflatable bag encircles the arm and the width is three quarters the length of the upper arm will give the most reliable readings and allow access of the stethoscope to the brachial artery. Korotkov phase V (disappearance of sounds) often does not occur in children and it is advisable to use muffling of sounds (phase IV) until after puberty. The child should be seated comfortably and quietly for several minutes and at least 3 measurements provided on any one occasion. Because of blood pressure variability it is likely that non-invasive ambulatory readings will be used increasingly to evaluate pressures in those considered at higher risk. Blood pressures recorded while children are agitated or distressed are likely to be elevated and every attempt should be made to repeat readings at a later stage. Except in severe and symptomatic cases decisions on management of those with raised pressures should only be made after readings have been repeated over a number of weeks.

What constitutes 'hypertension' in childhood?

As with adults, blood pressure levels are normally distributed in populations of children, with a skew deviation to the right. There is no sharp dividing line between normal and high blood pressure so that definitions of hypertension are purely arbitrary. High blood pressure in children is just that, ie. and a quantitative deviation from the norm which needs to take account of 'norms' for any given age and sex. The USA Second Task Force on Blood Pressure Control has suggested a classification into 'significant' or 'severe' hypertension according to the upper 3 and 1 percentiles in different age categories, taking into account the rapid rise in pressure in the first few weeks of life, the subsequent gradual increase until puberty, and the acceleration accompanying puberty and adolescence (Fig. 1). In the use of such definitions based on North American norms it is necessary to bear in mind that blood pressure levels in children vary considerably according to circumstances of measurement. As with adults, there is a marked effect of familiarization with repeated blood pressure readings so that values on a second or third occasion are substantially lower than the first. Blood pressure levels are also influenced by environmental temperature such that a 15°C temperature rise from 20 to 35°C can reduce pressures by 8–10 mmHg systolic and diastolic. Furthermore, the growth spurt of puberty which is accompanied by a rise in pressure can occur over a broad age range. Using the USA Task Force definitions for hypertension, 3% of children of 3–5 years of age would have systolic >112 or diastolic >76 mmHg and be labelled as having significant hypertension, and 1% would have figures of >124/>84, representing severe hypertension. By age 16–18 years, corresponding 'cut off' points are >142/>79 and >150/>98 respectively for 'significant' and 'severe' hypertension.

The problem with using these definitions is that of course the upper percentiles are 'high', and a proportion of the population must fall into these categories. The question is, do they matter?; i.e. do children with these levels of blood pressure have underlying pathology and are they predisposed to significant risk of cardiovascular disease? The answer is yes and no. The more severe the blood pressure elevation in childhood, the greater the likelihood that it reflects underlying renal or endocrine disease, and that the child is at risk of death or disability in the short term. Similarly the children with blood pressures in the third percentile are more likely to remain with high blood pressures and to develop clinically significant hypertension in adult life, while those with lower blood pressures are more likely to remain low. This is the phenomenon of so-called 'tracking', by which children tend to retain their 'ranking' for blood pressure levels, as they do for body weight, obesity and blood cholesterol levels. However, the strength of the correlation of blood pressures measured in children over 7-year periods is not so strong as to avoid a substantial proportion initially identified as 'hypertensive' being misclassified – while an even greater number of those regarded as 'normotensive' will subsequently become hypertensive. Two factors which may help to identify children most at risk of subsequent hypertension are obesity and family history. Obese children tend to have higher pressures and are more prone to become hypertensive as adolescents or adults if they gain excess weight. Similarly, children whose parents or siblings are hypertensive are more prone to have higher pressures, particularly where both parents, multiple siblings or twins are affected.

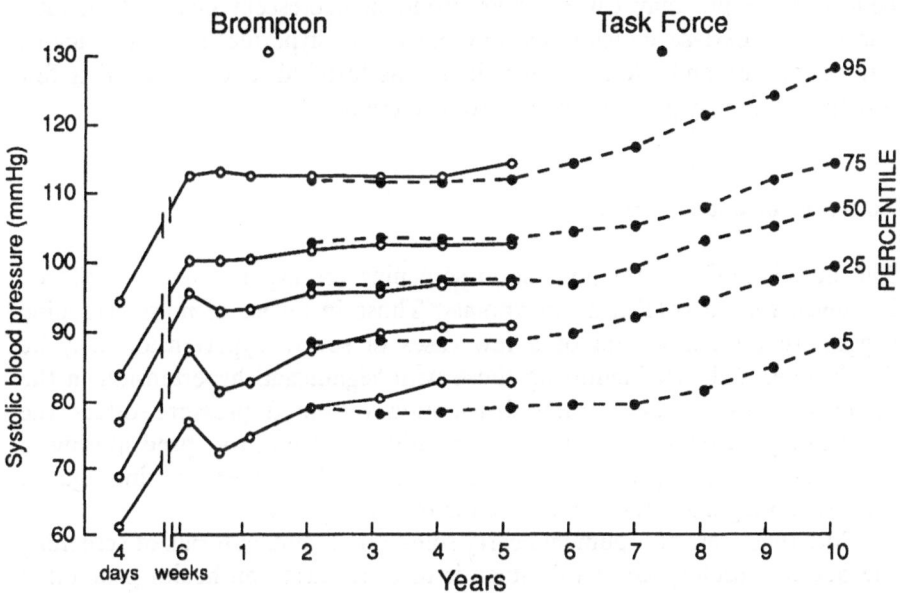

Fig. 1. Quintiles of blood pressures (systolic) in children in relation to age. Brompton data from: M. de Swiet *et al.* (1980): *Pediatrics* 65: 1028. Task force data from: S. Blumenthal *et al.* (1977): *Pediatrics* 59: 797

Severe symptomatic hypertension and secondary hypertension

Most of the children with significant or even severe hypertension as defined above have no obvious cause for the blood pressure elevation if it is detected by routine screening. In contrast, life-threatening hypertension in childhood and adolescence is normally symptomatic at an earlier stage than in adults, either from a specific underlying cause, or by virtue of hypertensive headaches, heart failure or fits. The commoner causes of symptomatic severe childhood hypertension in countries with good socio-economic conditions are chronic renal disease, in the form of chronic glomerulonephritis and chronic pyelonephritis due to reflux nephropathy, and renal artery stenosis which is often segmental in nature. In poorer countries acute glomerulonephritis tends to predominate. Underlying chronic renal disease frequently leads to stunted growth and fatigue. Other important but rarer causes of childhood hypertension are phaeochromocytoma, presenting as sustained hypertension or with characteristic paroxysmal symptoms or accompanying neurofibromatosis, primary aldosteronism, presenting with symptoms of weakness, polyuria, and/or tetany from hypokalaemia, and aortic coarction. Liquorice addiction may mimic primary aldosteronism and the oral contraceptive pill may cause hypertension in adolescent girls. Congenital adrenal hydroxylase deficiencies may present as hypertension in infancy or later childhood and excess sodium intake as fortified foods in the first few months of life may precipitate hypertensive crises.

To screen or not to screen?

The question of general population screening for hypertension in children has given rise to conflicting viewpoints. Those in favour of mass screening suggest that identification of a few cases of severe hypertension may be worthwhile, and that identifying those with 'significant' hypertension in the upper centiles of the normal distribution of blood pressure offers the opportunity for intervention to try to modify life-style factors predisposing to more severe blood pressure elevation in later life. Those arguing against mass screening make the points listed in the box opposite.

Both these sets of arguments carry some sense, and, in terms of screening the authors' preference at this stage is to concentrate on health promotion programmes for all children and avoid excessive 'labelling', but to screen those at highest risk in terms of a strong family history of blood pressure elevation and/or cardiovascular and renal disease and those children who are already overweight or who have disorders, such as neurofibromatosis, associated with hypertension. Further refinements in our ability to predict tracking of blood pressures may lead us to alter this approach.

ARGUMENTS AGAINST MASS SCREENING

* The cost of total child population screening is substantial for the very small yield of severe hypertensives.

* A significant proportion of those 'labelled' as hypertensives will be mislabelled. There are likely to be consequent costs and unnecessary anxiety.

* As most of the overall cardiovascular morbidity and mortality in the general population occurs in those in the upper half of the distribution of blood pressure levels, and, not the upper 1–3%, there is more to be gained by public health measures aimed at all children.

* Blood pressure is only one of a number of risk factors for cardiovascular disease and it would seem more logical to put limited resources into tackling physical fitness insufficiency, obesity, fat intake and smoking in children.

Management of the hypertensive child

Symptomatic and severe hypertension in childhood often has an identifiable cause. A comprehensive clinical and laboratory assessment will be necessary, evolving along lines suggested by initial leads as indicated above. Clinical examination will focus on evidence of enlarged kidneys, renal bruits, normal femoral pulses and leg pressures to exclude coarctation, signs of cardiac hypertrophy and heart failure, retinopathy, and adrenogenital syndromes.

In the absence of other clues all children who are hypertensive on repeated measurement will require assessment of mid-stream urine for cells, casts, bacteria, protein and sugar, plasma urea electrolytes and creatinine and chest X-ray, ECG and echo evidence of cardiac enlargement. Abdominal ultrasound will establish kidney size, masses, cysts and evidence of obstruction. In very severe or symptomatic cases, 24-hour urine catecholamines should be estimated and renal angiography used to exclude renal artery stenosis.

Hypertensive headaches, left ventricular failure or fits and severe hypertension associated with renal impairment will require immediate hospitalization and blood pressure reduction. Where possible, pressures should be lowered by oral therapy, with liquid nifedipine currently as first choice, but where this fails or the patient is vomiting or comatose carefully titrated intravenous diazoxide or hydralazine or intravenous sodium nitroprusside should be used with frequent blood pressure monitoring to avoid excessive hypotension.

The choice of drugs for oral maintenance therapy is as in the adult (Chapter 10), with a particular need to try to avoid centrally acting drugs which cause sedation or depression. Diuretics may be necessary in combination with other drugs to achieve adequate blood pressure control but in view of their long-term effects on glucose tolerance and lipid metabolism they should be avoided in milder cases. Drug regimes should be administered once daily where possible to simplify treatment and improve compliance.

Non-pharmacological approaches should be used in all cases with a view to reducing drug needs in more severe hypertension and avoiding therapy in those with milder hypertension in whom monitoring should be continued for several months before using drugs. Efforts should be concentrated on weight control and regular exercise. Dietary measures to reduce total and saturated fat intake and increase fruit and vegetable consumption will have the added benefits of reducing blood cholesterol levels. Sodium restriction appears to be less effective in children and adolescents than in elderly subjects, but may help potentiate the action of antihypertensive drugs and reduce the need for diuretic therapy. In acute glomerulonephritis with fluid retention, salt and water restriction will be mandatory.

Advice on avoidance of alcohol and smoking in hypertensive children and adolescents, and on maintaining ideal body weight should be part of the long-term programme. Careful counselling of children and parents will be necessary to ensure compliance with medical advice and treatment, with a view to ensuring full integration into normal childhood and adolescent activities and avoiding an excessive preoccupation with the concept of ill health.

PREGNANCY

Hypertension in pregnancy remains one of the principal causes of perinatal and maternal mortality and morbidity. Hypertensive pregnant women should be supervized in consultation with a specialist obstetric unit and a consultant physician with special experience of the problem. Patients should be delivered in hospitals with appropriate resuscitation facilities and immediate access to a neonatal paediatrician.

Hypertension in pregnancy may be a continuation of pre-existing hypertension, or occur as part of the complex syndrome of pre-eclampsia. The syndrome also comprises renal impairment, a disturbance of coagulation, platelet consumption, and, in its severe form, fits, and renal and liver failure. Fetal growth is often retarded and still-birth may occur in association with retroplacental haemorrhage. Pre-eclampsia is commoner in first pregnancies and frequently supervenes on pre-existing hypertension. An underlying disturbance of the immune relationship between fetus and mother may be the cause and the pathophysiology is thought to involve an imbalance between vasodilator prostacyclin production, which is suppressed, and excessive release of vasoconstrictor and pro-aggregatory thromboxane contributing to placental ischaemia and renal and systemic vasoconstriction.

Blood pressures normally fall early in pregnancy due to a profound systemic vasodilatation, disproportionately exceeding the rise in cardiac output (Fig. 2). Although blood pressure levels over 140/90 are arbitrarily designated hypertensive, levels over 130/80 before 20 weeks gestation should be regarded with suspicion. Pre-eclampsia should be suspected if there is a change in the rate of weight gain of the mother, impaired fetal growth, or a

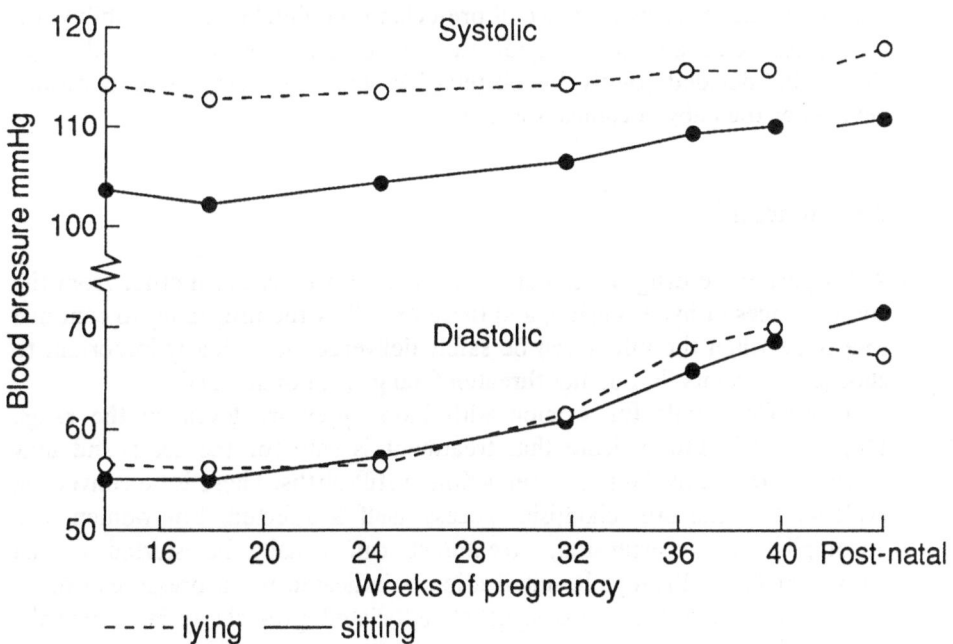

Fig. 2. Average blood pressure of 226 primiparae, measured using a London School of Hygiene sphygmomanometer to avoid observer bias. Reproduced by permission of *Clinical Science*: MacGillivray, Rose and Rowe (1969): 37:395

rising plasma rate or falling platelet count in a hypertensive pregnant woman. Development of proteinuria in uninfected urine is a serious sign of pre-eclampsia.

Assessment

Clinical and laboratory assessment of the condition of the mother should be as for the non-pregnant hypertensive but with avoidance of radiation until postpartum unless essential. Severe hypertensives should be examined carefully for evidence of heart failure and retinal haemorrhages exudates or papilloedema. Evidence of underlying renal tract infection and glomerulonephritis should be sought from the history and urine analysis. Renal ultrasound can exclude urinary tract obstruction and polycystic kidneys and avoids radiation exposure. Although phaeochromocytoma is rare, it is often fatal if undiagnosed in pregnancy, hence 24-hour urine should be analysed for catecholamines. Patients should be seen fortnightly by obstetricians and/or physicians for measurement of blood pressures (left lateral and standing) and weight; clinical assessment of fetal growth; mid-stream urine testing for protein and blood urea, creatinine, uric acid and platelet count for early evidence of pre-eclampsia. Fetal size and viability will be assessed clinically and by abdominal ultrasound. The timing of delivery should be decided jointly by obstetrician and physician if complications develop or the baby becomes overdue.

When to treat

Antihypertensive drug treatment is designed to protect the mother from the consequences of hypertension, and therefore allow the pregnancy to continue to a stage when the infant can be safely delivered. It is clearly important to choose treatments that do not threaten fetal growth or survival.

Controlled trials for women with blood pressure levels in the range 140/90 to 170/110 indicate that treatment is safe for the fetus and may improve fetal survival due to a reduction in still-births. There is no convincing evidence that the pre-eclampsia process itself is affected. For women with uncomplicated hypertension, treatment can usually be started on an outpatient basis. Prompt hospitalization is indicated when pressures exceed 170/110 or when there are signs of associated pre-eclampsia, especially proteinuria.

Choice of drugs

Drugs that have been subjected to controlled trials and appear to be safe for the fetus include α-methyldopa, β-blockers such as atenolol, alprenolol and labetalol, and clonidine. Drug doses, side-effects and mode of administration are as in the non-pregnant, although requirements may decrease in early pregnancy in women with pre-existing hypertension, and often increase again in late pregnancy, particularly if pre-eclampsia supervenes. α-Methyldopa has been subjected to the most rigorous controlled trials with one study commencing at the twelfth week of pregnancy and with follow-up of the offspring of treated mothers up to the age of 7 years. Methyldopa is rarely given long enough for haemolytic anaemia to develop, but sedation and postural faintness are common. β-Blockers appear to be better tolerated in pregnancy and to be safe for the fetus, although neonatal bradycardia and pallor is sometimes observed and may continue if mothers on high doses are breast feeding. Vasodilators such as hydralazine and the α-adrenoreceptor blocker, prazosin, can be combined with β-blockers or methyldopa in resistant cases, but the peripherally acting calcium-channel blockers such as nifedipine are becoming more commonly used in this situation. Verapamil is also effective but may delay the onset and progress of labour.

Antihypertensive drugs to be avoided in pregnancy are the angiotensin converting enzyme (ACE) inhibitors, which can cause a high incidence of still-births in animals. Dihydropyridine analogues such as nifedipine are teratogenic in animals and should be avoided in the first three months of pregnancy. Reserpine should be avoided in late pregnancy as it can cause severe fetal depression if given within three weeks of delivery. Adrenergic neurone drugs have generally been superseded by agents less prone to cause postural hypotension. The use of clonidine should be avoided because of the possibility of severe rebound hypertension if it is stopped suddenly. Diuretic therapy should be avoided except in congestive heart failure as plasma volume is low in hypertensive pregnancies, particularly with pre-eclampsia. Similarly there is no place for dietary sodium restriction in hypertensive pregnancies, even when oedema is present.

The risk of developing pre-eclampsia and losing the fetus increases in proportion to the severity of pre-existing hypertension. In women whose blood pressure is controlled on antihypertensive drugs and who are planning conception it is probably safer to continue treatment despite a small and often unknown risk of teratogenicity. The exception is with ACE inhibitors, where with current suspicions of their effects on fetal loss, it is preferable to change to an alternative agent before conceiving, or soon after if conception occurs while on these agents. Sometimes the vasodilatation of early pregnancy leads to low normal pressures (say less than 110/70) in women on antihypertensive drugs. In these circumstances doses may be cautiously reduced, and then re-instituted if necessary later in pregnancy. Frequent follow-up is of course essential if these steps are taken. Similarly, if blood pressure has been well controlled without side-effects on drugs other than those indicated as preferred treatments, it is probably best to continue that regime throughout pregnancy (ACE inhibitors, reserpine and diuretics excepted).

Prevention of pre-eclampsia

None of the antihypertensive drugs subject to controlled trials in mild hypertension in pregnancy have been shown to influence other features of pre-eclampsia. There have been no controlled trials in women with pressures >170/110, although uncontrolled series certainly suggest that treatment will allow pregnancies to continue to fetal viability that otherwise would have been terminated on the grounds of maternal risk alone. Recently there have been 3 controlled trials suggesting that relatively low-dose aspirin can prevent proteinuria, increase fetal growth and survival and reduce the incidence of severe pre-eclampsia in women with mild pre-eclampsia or at high risk of developing it. The mechanism is thought to be via inhibition of thromboxane synthesis. Further large-scale trials are in progress for what may be a most valuable adjunct to the management of this disorder.

Hypertensive emergencies in pregnancy

In addition to 'obstetric' indicators for hospitalization, urgent blood pressure reduction is indicated if hypertension is associated with symptoms of impending eclampsia, such as headaches, flashing lights or abdominal pain. Five drops (say) of oral nifedipine swallowed will often reduce pressures within 5 minutes and doses may be repeated as required every 10 minutes, up to a dose of 30 mg, and then at 2–3 hour intervals. For patients who are vomiting or are resistant to oral nifedipine, slow infusion of diazoxide (10 mg/min up to 300 mg) or 5 mg boluses of hydralazine are usually effective, but may cause throbbing headaches, palpitations, flushing and vomiting. They should be supplemented by oral β-blockers or methyldopa and the baby delivered by Caesarian section if the fetus is considered viable. Patients on pre-existing antihypertensive drugs are particularly sensitive to the hypotensive effect of intravenous vasodilators or liquid nifedipine.

In severe pre-eclampsia, blood pressure is often highest during the night and the timing of drug administration should take this into account.

Post partum

Antihypertensive therapy can usually be curtailed within a few days of delivery in 'pure' pre-eclampsia. However, occasionally there are transient exacerbations of severe hypertension and/or fits in the first week after delivery, and blood pressure may take a few weeks to subside. Persisting hypertension usually reflects pre-existing chronic hypertension the presence of which may have been masked by the vasodilatation of early pregnancy. All pregnant hypertensives should be carefully investigated for underlying causes of hypertension, and blood pressures should be monitored indefinitely in view of the increased risk of developing more severe hypertension in later life.

THE ELDERLY

Most doctors approach the management of the elderly hypertensive with a caution which is well justified, as, although the benefits of treatment can be high, there is a significant risk of doing more harm than good by injudicious decisions to treat, inappropriate use of drugs or inadequate monitoring of therapy.

The risks of hypertension

Hypertension is the major risk factor for stroke, heart failure and heart attack in the elderly. The risk rises progressively with increasing levels of systolic and diastolic blood pressure, at least up until 80 years of age. Systolic pressure is a better predictor of atherosclerotic brain infarction than diastolic pressure. The risk from isolated systolic pressure (defined as >160 mmHg with diastolic levels <90 mmHg) is also proportional to the height of the blood pressure. As cardiovascular disease accounts for >50% of deaths in the elderly and high blood pressure is common, the problem represents a major issue for medical management and public health.

Comparative figures on the prevalence of hypertension are strongly influenced by the circumstances of measurement and definition of hypertension. For example, following an initial blood pressure screening which has revealed a level of >160 mmHg systolic in an elderly subject, blood pressure may fall by 10 mmHg on a second visit, and will often continue to decline if readings are repeated over several weeks. Consequently, the estimated prevalence of hypertension in over 65-year-old defined by a cut off point of 160 mmHg systolic, will fall from about 45% to less than 10%.

Causes of hypertension in the elderly

As in younger subjects in most instances no clear-cut major disease process can be identified as the cause of hypertension in the elderly. However, most of the renal and endocrine disorders presenting in the younger age group may do so in older subjects and should be considered on clinical grounds at least, and in severe cases by further investigation. Atheromatous renal artery stenosis increases in frequency with ageing, and, if bilateral and severe, may be brought to light by the onset of renal failure if angiotensin II converting enzyme (ACE) inhibitors are given. Recent acceleration of hypertension with renal impairment in conjunction with a normal urine sediment and absence of prostate obstruction should also raise the suspicion of severe bilateral renal artery stenosis with occlusion of one renal artery. Abdominal bruits and an abdominal aortic aneurysm may be accompanying evidence of severe atherosclerosis.

Benign or malignant phaeochromocytoma is rare in the elderly but may present with characteristic symptoms of attacks of palpitations, throbbing headaches and tremor, sometimes associated with weight loss, diarrhoea or diabetes emeritus. Primary aldosteronism may persist undiagnosed from middle years into old age, until severe hypokalaemia becomes manifest, often in response to diuretic therapy. Thyrotoxicosis, hypothyroidism and hyperparathyroidism are all associated with hypertension, detection of which may be the first clue to their diagnosis. Chronic renal disease due to prostatic obstruction or low-grade chronic glomerulonephritis or pyelonephritis may underly hypertension in elderly subjects, and should be routinely sought by history clinical evaluation, mid-stream urine analysis and blood urea and creatinine estimations. Hypertension and diabetes mellitus are commonly associated, particularly in obese elderly subjects, and postprandial and/or fasting blood sugars should be checked before commencing treatment with and monitored while on, thiazide diuretic therapy.

Although the majority of cases labelled as 'primary' or essential hypertension will have no obvious underlying pathology, in many instances dietary or other life-style factors will be operating as in younger subjects. Excess body fat, regular alcohol consumption and a sedentary life style appear to be related to elevated blood pressure in a quantitative manner. Elderly subjects are also more susceptible to the pressor effect of a high salt intake, and hence stand to gain more by dietary sodium restriction than younger subjects. Non-steroidal anti-inflammatory drugs are used very widely, and often inappropriately, in the elderly, sometimes causing hypertension or antagonizing the effect of antihypertensive therapy.

Initial assessment

The following guidelines are suggested for subjects in the 65–80 year age range, although it is more sensible to base discussion on biological rather than chronological age in asymptomatic patients.

In addition to a carefull medical history detailed information should be obtained on drinking and smoking habits, ingestion of non-steroidal anti-inflammatory drugs and other prescribed and non-prescribed agents. Social background, psychological status and diet should be assessed, and where appropriate, evidence of dementia sought from the patient and relatives. This information is essential to enable the physician to evaluate the capacity of the patient to understand and comply with medical advice and regular drug therapy.

Clinical assessment (including history, examination and baseline investigations) should focus on common disorders in the elderly which may influence the decision to treat, the choice of drugs and the response to them. Evidence should be sought for cardiac ischaemia, diabetes, renal impairment, chronic lung disease and cerebrovascular and peripheral vascular disease, mood and gait disorders and thyroid disease.

Blood pressure should be measured over a number of weeks unless urgent therapy is indicated by cardiac failure, angina, accelerated or malignant hypertension or other hypertensive emergencies such as haemorrhagic stroke, aortic dissection or renal failure. Pressures should be measured using an appropriate cuff size with the patient sitting or supine and standing. Treatment should be based on the lower of the values to avoid symptomatic hypotension, or at the worst cerebral infarction. Pseudohypertension should be considered as mentioned above.

Baseline investigations for patients considered for treatment should include mid-stream urine microscopy and culture, blood creatinine and electrolytes, blood sugar and uric acid, liver function tests for evidence of heavy drinking, a blood count including mean corpuscular volume, electrocardiogram and chest X-ray. More expensive or invasive investigations for underlying causes of hypertension will depend not only on clinical suspicion and abnormal baseline tests, but on the likelihood that the results will materially influence management. Renal ultrasound will exclude severe urinary tract obstruction and may give useful information on the size and outline of the kidneys or the pressure of renal cysts, and has largely eliminated the need for intravenous pyelography for these purposes in the elderly.

Therapeutic approach

Blood pressure control has the potential to substantially improve both the quality and length of life. The extent to which this potential benefit can be realized has only been evaluated to a limited extent by controlled trials, but three studies in particular suggest that antihypertensive therapy leads to substantial reductions in morbidity. Both the Australian National Blood Pressure Study (entry diastolic 90 to 109 mmHg) and the American High Blood Pressure Detection Programme for 'stepped care' (specialist clinic) versus 'usual care' (practitioners) indicated a reduction of fatal and non-fatal strokes of around 45% in subjects over 60 years. The European Working Party on Hypertension in the Elderly (EWPHE) Trial involved a placebo-controlled study in 840 subjects aged 60 years or over with pressures > 160/90 mmHg and, according to the 'intention to treat' analysis, showed a 27% reduction in cardiovascular mortality and 38% fall in cardiac mortality with treatment. Ischaemic stroke and transient cerebral ischaemic rates also both fell substantially and overall there were 29 fewer cardiovascular events and 14 fewer cardiovascular deaths per 1000 patient years in treated versus placebo groups. As the 'event' rate is far higher in older than younger subjects the potential for prevention for the individual is correspondingly greater.

With this background we can then consider the special problems in relation to management of high blood pressure in older subjects.

When to treat?

In subjects who are symptomatic as a result of hypertensive left ventricular failure, associated angina or accelerated or malignant hypertension the decision to treat is relatively easy. In contrast, in relatively asymptomatic elderly subjects the decision to treat may depend principally on the level of blood pressure per se, and in these circumstances, unless the initial readings are exceptionally high, measurements should be repeated over a few weeks or in borderline cases 3 to 4 months. During this period of observation and assessment appropriate non-drug approaches to blood pressure control can be seriously attempted. On the basis of the limited trial data treatment should be instituted in asymptomatic patients whose pressures remain over 160 systolic or 100 diastolic. The more severe the hypertension the greater the risk and the earlier treatment should be started. In the case of severe hypertension, say >240 mmHg systolic and >120 mmHg diastolic with little postural fall, drugs should be started after 2 weeks or so.

Before considering therapy, blood pressures should always be measured in the standing position as well as the usual resting supine or seated readings in view of the greater tendency for postural hypotension in the elderly (see also Chapter 1). Postprandial hypotension is common and sometimes symptomatic in the elderly so that the timing of recent large meals may be relevant to the decision whether to treat and in the assessment of blood pressure control.

Practitioners should be aware of so called 'pseudohypertension' in which blood pressure is overestimated by standard non-invasive techniques due to excessively rigid arteries. It has been suggested that this may be anticipated by 'Osler's manoeuvre' which involves palpating the radial artery during temporary brachial artery occlusion. However, the sensitivity and specificity of this test is rather low, and other clues to falsely high pressure readings are the absence of echocardiographic evidence of left ventricular hypertrophy despite the presence of apparently high systolic pressures, or faintness following introduction antihypertensives in the absence of marked hypotension.

The decision when to treat elderly hypertensives depends very much on individual circumstances. Factors other than blood pressure levels that are likely to influence the decision to treat include cardiac, renal and cerebral impairment, other medical disorders, concomitant drug therapy and psychosocial factors.

Non-drug management (See also Chapter 7)

Subjects with sustained diastolic pressures over 100 mmHg and systolic levels more than 160 mmHg appear to benefit from blood pressure reduction by drugs, but in the absence of any urgent need for blood pressure reduction it is advisable to commence with non-pharmacological approaches as in younger patients, including, when appropriate, weight reduction, alcohol moderation to a maximum of two standard drinks a day, restriction of dietary salt, and gently graded aerobic exercise in the form of walking, cycling or swimming. Dietary advice aimed at calorie restriction should emphasize a reduction in saturated fat and an increase in fruit and vegetable consumption, taking care to maintain an adequate intake of essential nutrients, minerals and vitamins, especially for patients on a low income or socially isolated. If non-steroidal anti-inflammatory drugs are being used for pain relief for osteoarthritis, paracetamol should be tried as an alternative. Over-the-counter preparations containing sympathomimetic amines may cause hypertensive crises and should be avoided. These non-pharmacological measures may enable patients to avoid antihypertensive drugs or minimise their use.

The hazards of smoking continue into old age and stopping smoking is likely to delay the onset of coronary, cerebral and peripheral vascular disease and to reduce the risk of respiratory disorders. However, blood pressure tends to rise after smoking cessation, principally due to the tendency to gain weight.

Careful explanation, education and reassurance of elderly hypertensives and their families is even more important for long-term management than in the young.

Drug treatment (See also Chapter 8)

Drug treatment should be considered in symptomatic or severely hypertensive patients, or when blood pressures in asymptomatic hypertensives remain elevated over 3–6 months despite an adequate trial of non-pharmacological approaches. Exceptions to the use of drug therapy in asymptomatic hypertensives would include severe dementia, terminal disease, and some cases of severly incapacitating stroke. The higher the pressures, including systolic pressure, and the greater the evidence of cardiac or renal damage, the sooner treatment should be started.

Although many elderly hypertensives will truly lack symptoms others will have previously experienced stroke, cardiac or respiratory problems or claudication, and knowledge of the particular hazards of different types of antihypertensive drugs in these situations will help steer the physician and patient away from trouble. Therapy should be tailored carefully for every individual to minimize the risk of side-effects.

Responses to drug therapy can be affected by age-related falls in renal function, decreased plasma volume, and altered liver function, all of which can lead to increased circulating drug levels. Drug-induced postural blood pressure falls are likely to be exacerbated as a result of decreased cardiac output, impaired baroreceptor function and autonomic neuropathy. These postural effects are often further complicated by drugs given for other disorders, e.g. by digitalis or psychotropic agents and by increased susceptibility to volume depletion.

Antihypertensive therapy may unmask disorders commonly associated with hypertension such as myocardial ischaemia and impaired contractility, congestive heart failure and conduction defects leading to severe bradycardia and syncope. In the presence of severe stenoses affecting the coronary, cerebral, renal or peripheral circulation, blood pressure reduction and/or reduced cardiac output may precipitate or aggravate angina, cerebral ischaemia and infarction, renal failure and intermittent claudication.

A variety of other disorders occur with increased frequency with ageing and may influence the response to different types of antihypertensive drugs, e.g. chronic lung disease, diabetes mellitus, gout, depression, dementia, gait

92

disturbances and malnutrition. The ability or motivation to understand and comply with therapy may be further affected by visual impairment, deafness, isolation, poverty and in the case of immigrants, language difficulties. As any antihypertensive drug may cause a precipitous fall in blood pressure in elderly subjects the following points are essential:

RULES OF THUMB FOR OLDER HYPERTENSIVES

* Start with smaller doses, at most half the standard younger adult dose.

* Increase doses far more gradually – over several weeks.

* Titrate doses against standing pressures to avoid excessive orthostatic hypotension

* Avoid as first choice of therapy drugs particularly prone to cause orthostatic hypotension (prazosin, methyldopa, labetalol).

* Try to use simple, once-daily, regimes to improve compliance.

* Avoid centrally depressing drugs (clonidine, methyldopa, reserpine) which may lead to depression, confusion or pseudodementia.

* Monitor renal function and electrolyte status in patients on diuretics and/or ACE inhibitors.

Small doses of diuretics are often effective in the elderly, but patients are more prone to metabolic abnormalities such as changes in potassium, glucose intolerance and renal impairment. ACE inhibitors, either alone or in combination with diuretics will suit many patients, and generally lack central nervous depressing effects. They are particularly suitable for patients with coincident heart failure. Irritating cough may be troublesome. ACE inhibitors predispose to potassium retention by suppressing aldosterone release and should not usually be given with potassium sparing diuretics or potassium supplements. Non-steroidal anti-inflammatory drugs, β-blockers and renal impairment can all enhance this tendency to hyperkalaemia. As mentioned previously ACE inhibitors may precipitate renal failure in patients with bilateral renal artery stenosis, or stenosis in a single functioning kidney. Calcium-channel blockers are generally effective in the elderly. Verapamil is more prone to cause constipation in older subjects and may precipitate heart failure in those with pre-existing heart disease. The peripherally acting calcium-channel blockers such as nifedipine and felodipine act predominantly as arteriolar vasodilators and may aggravate angina by causing a reflex tachycardia. They may also give rise to gravitational oedema, flushing and headaches.

β-Blockers are often effective in the elderly although tiredness is poorly tolerated. Exacerbation of chronic airways disease, or claudication, or precipitation of heart failure is more likely to be seen because of the increased frequency of these disorders. Again judicious selection of the right drugs for the individual will enable most of these problems to be avoided.

Combinations of antihypertensive drugs will have additive or synergistic effects as in younger subjects; however, the risks of side-effects will also multiply, and problems of compliance increase the more complex the regimes.

The above discussion has centred around management of hypertensive patients up to 80 years of age. For older subjects who are symptomatic or already on antihypertensive therapy the same principles apply. However, the use of antihypertensive drug therapy for the very elderly patient without symptoms is questionable as a preventative measure.

The issue raises interesting philosophical and ethical questions as regards the objectives and costs of preventive medicine. However we can reflect that 20 years ago similar questions were posed in relation to those over 65 years of age. As the elderly become healthier and mentally and physically younger and as drug therapy improves, our approach to treatment may change correspondingly.

Selected references

Children
Report of the Second Task Force on Blood Pressure Control in Children (1987): *Pediatrics* 79: 1–25.
Clarke WR, Schrott HG, Leaverton PF, Connor WE, Laver RM (1978): Tracking of blood lipids and blood pressures in school age children. The Muscatine Study. *Circulation* 58: 626–634.

Pregnancy
Cunningham FG, Gant NF (1989): Prevention of pre-eclampsia – A reality? *N. Engl J Med* 321: 606–607.
Redman CWG, Beilin LJ, Bonnar J, Ounsted NK (1976): Fetal outcome in trial of antihypertensive treatment in pregnancy. *Lancet* 2: 753–756.

Redman CWG, Beilin LJ, Bonnar J, Wilkinson RH (1976): Plasma urate measurement in predicting fetal death in hypertensive pregnancy. *Lancet* 1: 1370.
Rubin PC (1988): Treatment of hypertension in pregnancy. In: Handbook of Hypertension (Series Editors WH Birkenhäger, JL Reid). Volume 10 Hypertension in Pregnancy (Ed. PC Rubin). Elsevier, Amsterdam & New York.
Sibai BM (1988): Pitfalls in diagnosis and management of pre-eclampsia. *Am J Obstet Gynecol* 159 (1): 1–5.
Walters BNJ, Redman CWG (1984): Treatment of severe pregnancy associated hypertension with a calcium antagonist nifedipine. *Br J Obstet Gynaecol* 91: 330–336.

Elderly
Amery A, Birkenhäger W, Brixko P, Bulpitt C, Clement D, Deruytterre M, de Sachaepdryver A, Dollery C, Fagard R, Forette F *et al.* (1985): Mortality and morbidity results from the European Working Party on High Blood Pressure in the Elderly Trial. *Lancet* 1: 1349–1354.
Australian National Blood Pressure Study Management Committee (1980): The Australian therapeutic trial in mild hypertension. *Lancet* 1: 1261–1267.
Beilin LJ (1988): Editorial Review: The Fifth Sir George Pickering Memorial Lecture – Epitaph to Essential Hypertension – A preventable disorder of known aetiology? *J Hypertension* 6: 85–94.
Hypertension Detection and Follow-up Programme Cooperative Group. (1979): Five-year findings of the hypertension detection and follow-up programme. II. Mortality by race, sex and age. *J Am Med Assoc* 242: 2572–2577
Kannel WB (1986): Prevalence, incidence and hazards of hypertension in the elderly. *Am Heart J* 112(6): 1362–1363.
Kannel WB, Sotlie P (1975): Hypertension in Framingham. In: Epidemiology and Control of Hypertension (Ed. P Oglesby) Stratton Intercontinental Medical Book Corporation, New York, pp. 553–555.
Schoenberger JA (1986): Epidemiology of systolic and diastolic systemic blood pressure elevation in the elderly. *Am J Cardiol* 57: 45C–51C.

CHAPTER 6

How to deal with secondary hypertension

FRANS BOOMSMA, FRANS H.M. DERKX, ARIE J. MAN IN 'T VELD,
ANTON H. VAN DEN MEIRACKER and GERT J. WENTING

In this chapter the main types of secondary hypertension will be reviewed:

* Renovascular hypertension
* Pheochromocytoma
* Mineralocorticoid excess (Primary aldosteronisms)

RENOVASCULAR HYPERTENSION

Definition

Renovascular hypertension is the most common form of secondary hypertension and is caused by obstruction of a renal artery or one of its branches. The hypertension is due to increased secretion of renin by the affected kidney into the circulation. The biological end-product of the renin–angiotensin system is angiotensin II. Angiotensin II is a potent vasoconstrictor; it stimulates aldosterone secretion via the adrenal gland and enhances sympathetic nervous system activity. The radiographic demonstration of a stenosis in the renal vasculature does not automatically imply a causative relationship to concurrent hypertension. Autopsy studies have shown that up to 30% of patients with normal blood pressure have some degree of renal artery stenosis. On the other hand patients with long-standing *essential* hypertension may develop atherosclerotic obstructive disease of the renal vasculature. Renovascular hypertension is therefore defined as occlusive disease of the renal arteries that is cured by correction of the lesion, i.e. after technically adequate transluminal percutaneous renal angioplasty (PTRA), surgical correction or nephrectomy. Correction of the obstruction in the renal artery in a patient with essential hypertension will of course not cure high blood pressure.

Prevalence, pathophysiology and causes

The prevalence of renovascular hypertension in the general hypertensive population is not known. In referral centres the prevalence is estimated as 1–5%.

The causes of renovascular hypertension are summarized below.

CAUSES OF RENOVASCULAR HYPERTENSION

* Atherosclerotic lesions
* Fibromuscular dysplasia
* Emboli and thrombi
* External compression of renal artery
* Aneurysm
* Arteritis: polyarteritis nodosa, Takayashu disease

The percentage reduction in the diameter of the lumen of the renal artery stimulating the renin–angiotensin system and causing hypertension has been estimated to be more than 60%.

Atherosclerotic plaques most commonly occur in the proximal third of the renal artery, although plaques in the wall of the aorta may also obstruct the entrance of the renal artery. The presence of a post-stenotic dilatation, extensive vascular collateral circulation and/or a small kidney are all evidence for a clinically significant stenosis. Bilateral renal artery stenosis occurs in about one third of the cases of renovascular hypertension. If untreated there is a high probability for complete occlusion to occur in due time.

Fibromuscular dysplasia is characterized by a 'string-of-beads' appearance in the renal artery due to thickening of the media interspersed with aneurysmal dilatations in the distal two thirds of the renal artery, often extending into the segmental vessels. Histologically the fibromuscular dysplasias are divided into intimal, medial and periarterial dysplasia. Up to 95% is caused by the medial

98

type. There is a predilection for young women; the lesions are not confined to the renal arteries but may also occur in the carotid, cerebral and iliac arteries. In contrast to arteriosclerotic lesions, progression to complete obstruction seldom occurs.

Other causes of renal artery stenosis are rare. Examples are: external compression by haematoma, an anomalous muscular or fibrotic band, or a cyst.

Clinical features

In most cases hypertension is an asymptomatic condition and there are no clinical signs that can reliably distinguish renovascular hypertension from essential hypertension. Some clinical features, though, may suggest the presence of renovascular hypertension (below).

CLINICAL CLUES FOR THE DIAGNOSIS OF RENOVASCULAR HYPERTENSION

* Duration of hypertension shorter and severity more pronounced than that of essential hypertension.
* Abrupt onset of hypertension at any age.
* Worsening of previously well-controlled hypertension.
* Association with coronary heart disease, cerebrovascular disease and intermittent claudication.
* Rare in black hypertensives.
* History of smoking, both in arteriosclerotic and fibromuscular dysplasia.
* Physical examination: continuous systolic–diastolic abdominal bruit.
* Retinopathies (haemorrhages, exudates and papilloedama) are more common.
* Proteinuria is not uncommon.
* Elevated serum creatinine.
* Increase in serum creatinine during converting enzyme inhibitor therapy.
* Hypokalaemia is rare.

Screening and diagnostic tests

The diagnostic work-up in patients with suspected renovascular hypertension involves two major steps. The first is the anatomic demonstration of the obstruction by angiography. The second step is to prove whether or not the obstruction is the cause of hypertension and whether or not it could be cured by PTRA or surgery.

Radiographic vizualization is the only reliable method for demonstrating an obstruction in the renal artery or its main branches. However, angiography cannot be performed routinely in all patients with high blood pressure because this investigation is invasive and expensive. The following screening tests maximize the chances of finding a lesion by subsequent angiography in patients with clinical clues for renovascular hypertension:

1. Rapid-sequence intravenous pyelography (IVP)

The criteria for a positive test are:

a) A delayed appearance by more than one minute of the radiocontrast in the pelvic calyceal region of the affected kidney,
b) An increase in the concentration on the affected side 10–20 min after injection of the dye and
c) A smaller kidney size by at least 1.5 cm.

About 80% of patients with renal artery stenosis have one or more of these criteria, although false positive results are found in up to 15–20% of patients with essential hypertension. Other studies have shown that up to 50% of surgically cured patients had a normal IVP. Patients with bilateral stenosis also tend to present with a non-diagnostic IVP.

Other kidney diseases that are associated with hypertension such as pyelonephritis, urinary tract obstruction, polycystic disease and renal tumours, may also be discovered through the IVP.

2. Intravenous digital subtraction renal angiography

This method is less invasive than the arteriogram because the contrast medium is injected into a peripheral or a central vein. The method has, however, some major disadvantages, such as insufficient resolution, inadequate vizualization of the main branches of the renal artery and a relatively high dose of the radiocontrast substance required for imaging.

100

Moreover, the diagnostic value of the test is probably no better than that of IVP. Intravenous digital subtraction renal angiography at present is not advocated as a screening test for renovascular hypertension.

3. Renal scintigraphy

Radionuclide imaging techniques can provide valuable information regarding renal blood flow, excretory functions and renal perfusion–excretion ratios. ^{99m}Technecium diethylenetriamine penta-acetic acid (^{99m}Tc-DPTA) can be used as a measure of glomerular filtration rate, and with the development of computerized scintilation techniques it is also possible to image the kidney. ^{99m}Tc-DTPA has replaced the classical renogram and is used for both quantitative and qualitative functional assessment of the affected and non-affected kidney. The discriminative power of ^{99m}Tc-DTPA scintigraphy is increased by applying angiotensin converting enzyme therapy.

The following tests are advocated to prove whether or not the stenosis is the true cause of the hypertension.

4. Plasma renin activity (PRA)

The PRA test measures the rate of angiotensin I generation *in vitro* and is a measure of the renin concentration in plasma. The peripheral vein level of PRA can be regarded as a measure of renal secretion of renin. If PRA is determined under strictly standardized conditions and indexed against sodium excretion, about 50% of patients with renovascular hypertension have elevated PRA levels. However, up to 15% of patients with essential hypertension also have elevated renin levels. A casual measurement of PRA is therefore of little diagnostic value.

5. Captopril–renin test

Renovascular hypertensives with normal peripheral vein renin levels have an abnormal increase in plasma PRA to various stimuli such as sodium depletion, upright posture and administration of an angiotensin converting enzyme inhibitor (ACEI). Captopril was the first available angiotensin converting enzyme inhibitor. The time to reach peak levels of captopril after an oral dose is about 0.5–1.5 hours. The release of renin by the juxtaglomerular cell of the kidney is inhibited by angiotensin II and this negative feed-back mechanism is interupted by the ACEI. The discriminative power of a peripheral vein PRA is improved when blood samples are taken 1–2 hours after stimulation of renin by a single (first) dose of captopril.

6. Differential renal vein renin determination

This test has emerged as a useful test in identifying correctable renovascular hypertension. Under normal conditions the renal vein-to-artery ratio for renin is 1.25. A renal vein-to-artery renin ratio of 1.5 is considered to be elevated. An elevated renal vein-to-artery renin ratio on the affected side is caused by a diminished renal blood flow rather than an increase in renin secretion. A high renin ratio on the affected side and a suppressed ratio contralaterally is considered to predict a favourable surgical outcome.

Clinical management of renovascular hypertension

The objectives of percutaneous transluminal renal angioplasty or surgery are to prevent complications of hypertension by controlling blood pressure and to delay any (further) loss of renal function. The medical treatment of renovascular hypertension uses the same principles as the treatment of essential hypertension. There are no prospective studies available today comparing the long-term benefits and risks of surgical reconstruction or PTRA and pharmacological treatment.

Percutaneous transluminal renal angioplasty provides a non-surgical method for treating renal artery stenosis. The overall cure rate for renovascular hypertension is about 25% and 40% of patients are improved. Therefore about one third of patients will not benefit from this therapy. The method is, however, advocated in patients with fibromuscular dysplasia, because here the cure rate is about 50% as compared with 19% in patients with atherosclerotic disease. **Nephrectomy** was the first successful procedure for treating renovascular hypertension. With reconstructive surgery it is now possible to perform **bypass procedures** with autologous or synthetic grafts. The incidence of graft occlusion or restenosis following renal revascularization is low. Atherosclerotic lesions are progressive and if untreated may lead to end-stage renal failure. Therefore angioplasty or revascularization should be considered for the preservation of renal function even in the absence of hypertension. **Pharmacotherapy** with drugs that block the renin–angiotensin system can effectively control hypertension in most patients with renovascular hypertension. Patients with a severe unilateral stenosis and patients with bilateral stenosis must be monitored carefully because blood pressure control can be accompanied by loss of renal function.

Therapy should be stopped or changed if kidney function deteriorates. Patients on ACEI therapy should be especially monitored for loss of renal function not only by, measuring serum creatinine, but also by performing ^{99m}Tc-DTPA scintigraphy within one week after starting therapy, because in patients with unilateral stenosis, glomerular filtration in the affected kidney may fall to zero without significantly affecting serum creatinine. It should be borne in mind that alternative drugs (β-blockers, calcium antagonists) are likely to be effective and less hazardous when it comes to maintaining glomerular filtration pressure.

PHEOCHROMOCYTOMA

Definition

A pheochromocytoma is a tumour of chromaffin cells of neuroectodermal origin. Pheochromocytomas are mainly found in the adrenal gland, but they may be located throughout the sympathetic nervous system from the glomus jugulare to the urinary bladder.

SITES OF PHEOCHROMOCYTOMA

Site	Percentage
Abdominal	>97%
Adrenal	80–90%
– unilateral	80%
– bilateral	10%
Extra-adrenal*	10–20%
Extra-abdominal	<3%
Thoracic	<2%
Neck	<2%

* Common sites: lumbar-paravertebral, organ of Zuckerland, bladder, para-aortic.

Lesions arising outside the adrenal medulla are classified as extra-adrenal pheochromocytomas or functional paragangliomas. Ninety percent of pheochromocytomas are unilateral and sporadic, whereas the remaining 10% are multiple and/or familial. Unilateral or bilateral pheochromocytoma is the sole manifestation in half of the familial cases, whereas, in the other half, pheochromocytomas may be associated with familial endocrine tumour syndromes, such as multiple endocrine neoplasia (MEN) type IIa (medullary carcinoma of thyroid, hyperparathyroidism and pheochromocytoma) and MEN type IIb (medullary carcinoma of thyroid, mucosal neuromas, thickened corneal nerves, pheochromocytoma and frequently a Marfan-like habitus). Pheochromocytoma may also occur in association with neurofibromatosis (von Recklinghausen's disease). The incidence of a pheochromocytoma in this disorder is less than 1%, whereas the incidence of neurofibromatosis in patients with a pheochromocytoma is 5%. Rarely, pheochromocytoma coexists with von Hippel–Lindau disease (cerebellar haemangioblastoma and retinal angioma). About 10% of pheochromocytomas are malignant. Since histological differentiation is of no value, the criterium of malignancy is based on the presence of distant metastases.

Pathophysiology

The pathophysiology of pheochromocytomas is primarily related to the secretion of excessive amounts of catecholamines. The chromaffin cells synthesize catecholamines from the amino-acid precursor, tyrosine, with noradrenaline as the end product, except within the adrenal medulla where about 75% of noradrenaline is methylated to adrenaline. Consequently, most adrenal medullary pheochromocytomas secrete at least some adrenaline, whereas paragangliomas, if functional, only secrete noradrenaline. The secretion of catecholamines by pheochromocytomas varies considerably. Small tumours tend to secrete a larger proportion of active catecholamines, whereas larger tumours, owing to their capacity to store and metabolize large quantities of catecholamines, tend to secrete less of their contents and most of those in inactive forms.

Signs and symptoms

Most patients are symptomatic. Common symptoms are headache, palpitations, with or without tachycardia, and excessive and inappropriate sweating. Less commonly observed symptoms are anxiety, nervousness, tremulousness, facial pallor, nausea, weakness, fatigue and weight loss. In up to 50% of patients with pheochromocytoma, hypertension and symptoms occur in paroxysms, with normotensive symptom-free intervals between attacks. During attacks spectacular increments in blood pressure can occur. The paroxysms vary in frequency, duration and severity and are usually abrupt in onset but subside more slowly. In most patients they last less than one hour. Attacks may occur several times a month or several times a day. They may occur spontaneously or be precipitated by pressure in the region of the tumour, exercise, micturition, ingestion of food or beverages containing tyramine (e.g. ripe cheese, beer or wine), administration of certain drugs (e.g. histamine, glucagon, tyramine, phenothiazines, metoclopramide), intubation, anaesthesia, or operative manipulation. The features of an attack may suggest a number of other conditions. In the differential diagnosis, anxiety with hyperventilation, hypoglycaemia, angina pectoris, myocardial infarction, acute pulmonary oedema, migraine and cluster headaches, brain tumour, stroke, carcinoid, porphyria, lead poisoning and the clonidine withdrawal syndrome should be considered. To complicate matters further, paroxysms with or without very high blood pressures may lead to angina, myocardial infarction or acute pulmonary oedema. Of particular importance are recurrent symptoms of orthostatic hypotension. The mechanisms involved may be desensitization of adrenergic receptors, a depression of the sympathetic reflex response to upright posture and a reduced blood volume.

Diagnosis

1. Plasma and urinary catecholamines and metabolites

Measurement of plasma catecholamines and urinary catecholamines or their metabolites is a useful initial test for the detection of a pheochromocytoma. In patients with a proven pheochromocytoma, plasma catecholamines are almost always elevated. Reliable techniques for measuring plasma catecholamines are now widely available and are used with increasing frequency for the diagnosis. In order to prevent false positive results as much as possible, it is essential that blood is sampled under strictly basal conditions (intravenous cannula in situ, blood sampling after a supine rest period of 30 minutes). Determination of urinary vanillylmandelic acid excretion is still an ingrained method used for primary screening, although urinary catecholamines and/or (nor)-metanephrine levels are usually reported to be more specific and sensitive.

2. Clonidine suppression test

In subjects with elevated plasma catecholamines, in whom a pheochromocytoma cannot be detected by one of the localization techniques, the clonidine test may be helpful. Clonidine is a centrally acting α-adrenergic agonist which inhibits peripheral sympathetic outflow. The test is based on the principle that increases in plasma catecholamines are normally mediated through activation of the sympathetic nervous system, whereas, in patients with a pheochromocytoma, the elevations result from diffusion of excess catecholamines from the lesion into the circulation, bypassing normal storage and release mechanisms. Therefore clonidine should not be expected to suppress the release of catecholamines in patients with pheochromocytoma, whereas its administration to subjects without a pheochromocytoma should invariably lead to a fall in plasma catecholamines. In clinical practice, blood samples for measurement of catecholamines are taken before and 1, 2 and 3 hours after the oral administration of 0.3 mg of clonidine.

3. Glucagon stimulation test

If suspicion of a pheochromocytoma is high but determinations of plasma or urinary catecholamines remain equivocal, a pharmacological stimulation test can be performed. Glucagon is currently in use because of its relatively few side-effects. It is given as an i.v. bolus injection of 1.0 mg. In patients with a pheochromocytoma, glucagon may provoke arrhythmias and large increases in blood pressure. It is therefore mandatory that both ECG and blood pressure are monitored continuously. In addition syringes with phentolamine and propranolol should be ready for immediate use. It should be noted that in subjects without a pheochromocytoma, glucagon administration can also provoke a considerable rise in plasma adrenaline (Table 1).

In conjunction with the rise in adrenaline an increase in heart rate of about ten beats per minute and a small rise in systolic blood pressure is frequently observed. It should be borne in mind that nausea, sometimes with vomiting, regularly occurs.

Localization

A pheochromocytoma may be detected by various non-invasive techniques, including sonography, computerized axial tomography, MRI scanning and ^{123}I or ^{131}I-MIBG scintigraphy. These techniques have obviated the need for (potentially hazardous) arteriography. Since computerized tomography is extremely accurate in revealing adrenal lesions with a diameter as small as 1 cm, and since the majority of pheochromocytomas are to be found in the adrenal gland, it is the procedure of first choice for localizing a pheochromocytoma. The use of the radiopharmaceutical agents [131]I- or ^{123}I-metaiodobenzylguanidine (^{131}I, ^{123}I-MIBG) provides a relatively new technique for the diagnosis as well as the localization of pheochromocytomas. MIBG is an analogue of noradrenaline and has the propensity to become concentrated in chromaffin cell tumours. The uptake of ^{131}I-MIBG is quite variable and up to 15% of pheochromocytomas escape detection by this technique. MIBG scintigraphy is however useful for the detection of extra-adrenal and metastatic disease where computerized tomography may be less successful.

Table 1. Baseline values of plasma noradrenaline, adrenaline and dopamine and their response to glucagon, 1 mg i.v., in the absence or presence of a pheochromocytoma

	Absence of pheochromocytoma (*n* = 15)		*Presence of pheochromocytoma* (*n* = 5)	
	Baseline mean (range) pg/ml	*Glucagon response* mean (range) pg/ml	*Baseline* mean (range) pg/ml	*Glucagon response* mean (range) pg/ml
Noradrenaline	294 (84 – 442)	27 (–21 – 102)	635 (271 – 906)	6770 (250 – 14000)
Adrenaline	78 (21 – 176)	86 (4 – 142)	289 (105 – 528)	2320 (700 – 4000)
Dopamine	17 (6 – 46)	–2 (–12 – 3)	53 (16 – 86)	45 (2 – 120)

Medical treatment

Although surgical removal of the tumour is the ultimate remedy, preoperative treatment with an α-adrenergic blocking agent is almost always required in order to control symptoms, to re-expand plasma volume, and to minimize blood pressure fluctuations during introduction to anaesthesia and throughout the operation.

Phenoxybenzamine (Dibenzyline[R]), a long-acting moderately selective α_1-blocker is most commonly used. It is usually given in a twice-daily dose of 10–20 mg. Frequent side-effects of this drug are orthostatic hypotension, sedation and nasal stuffiness. Alternatives to phenoxybenzamine are the more selective α_1-blockers, prazosin, doxazosin or urapidil, but experience with these drugs in patients with pheochromocytoma is still limited.

β-Adrenoceptor blocking agents are also frequently given. Specific indications for their administration are supraventricular tachycardia and other arrhythmias. β-Blockers should never be given before blockade of α-adrenoceptors is established, since β-blockade *per se* may cause marked elevations in blood pressure. Blood pressure elevations are more pronounced with non-selective than with β_1-selective β-blockers because the former block vasodilatory β_2-receptors. Therefore β_1-selective blockers, like atenolol or metoprolol, are preferred over non-selective β-blockers like propranolol or nadolol. Labetolol, an agent with both α- and β-adrenoceptor blocking properties, has also been reported to be effective in preventing the symptoms of a pheochromocytoma. However, since its profile of α- and β-adrenoceptor antagonism is the reverse of what is theoretically required, we advice caution with respect to prescribing this drug in patients with a pheochromocytoma.

α-Methylparatyrosine (metyrosine, Demser[R]) blocks the synthesis of catecholamines by competitive inhibition of tyrosine hydroxylase. It is available in capsules of 250 mg and is usually administered in a dose of 250–1000 mg four times a day. It can be used as an alternative to or in addition to standard therapy with α-adrenergic blocking drugs. Because the bulk of the drug is excreted in the urine and since the amino acid is relatively insoluble in water, renal crystalluria is a potential hazard. Hence, water intake during the use of metyrosine should be maintained at an adequate level.

The short-acting non-selective α-blocker, phentolamine (Regitine[R]), with an initial dose of 2–5 mg followed by repeat injections or a constant infusion of 1 mg/min), and/or sodium nitroprusside (0.5–1.5 μg kg min^{-1} initially) are given to manage hypertensive crises that may arise during induction of anaesthesia, intubation and surgical manipulation of the tumour.

Surgery

Since induction of anaesthesia and surgery may be associated with hypertensive crises despite pretreatment with α-blockers, both ECG and arterial pressure should be monitored continuously. Rises in blood pressure during surgery are managed by i.v. infusions of phentolamine and nitroprusside. In the vast majority of patients the tumour is located in one of the adrenals, and, given the precision with which these tumours can nowadays be located before surgery, an abdominal approach is no longer necessary but an appropriate loin incision will suffice. With tumours outside the adrenals but within the abdominal cavity, and with bilateral lesions as in the familial syndromes, the abdominal approach is to be preferred. Hypotension, which may occur on clamping the tumour vessels on removal of the gland, is usually sufficiently treated by judicious volume replacement with plasma or blood. Sometimes, however, when hypotension is severe, an i.v. noradrenaline infusion (infusion rate 0.1–1.0 μg kg min^{-1}) has to be given as well. It is essential that the infusions are reduced gradually.

Malignant pheochromocytoma

Malignant pheochromocytomas usually follow an indolent course. Surgical debulking of tumour load takes precedence, since tumours and metastases are not very sensitive to radiation or chemotherapy. Manifestations due to excessive catecholamines are managed by medical treatment. Radiotherapy often temporarily controls the local symptoms of metastases. For disseminated disease, combination chemotherapy may give objective and subjective improvement in over 50% of patients. With the provision that ^{131}I-MIBG is concentrated by the tumour, high doses (100–200 mCi) of this agent may reduce tumour size and sometimes produce long-lasting improvement of symptoms in patients with disseminated disease.

MINERALOCORTICOID AND OTHER STEROID CAUSES OF HYPERTENSION

Introduction

The various causes of endocrine hypertension are listed overleaf.

Most of these entities are extremely rare and therefore the use of appropriate diagnostic tests should be dictated only by strong (expert) clinical suspicion. For practical purposes we focus on primary aldosteronism because of its relative frequency.

Primary aldosteronism

Excessive and relatively autonomous production of aldosterone (as a result of either adrenal adenoma or hyperplasia) appears to be the cause of hypertension in less than 0.5% of patients. Nevertheless, its recognition is important because hypertension associated with an adrenal adenoma can be cured. Unilateral adrenalectomy may spare the patient a lifetime of taking drugs. Primary aldosteronism is most prevalent between the ages of 30 and 40 and more common in females. Aldosterone-producing adenoma in particular is seen more often in women (2:1).

TYPES OF ENDOCRINE HYPERTENSION

* Primary aldosteronism
  - adenoma
  - bilateral hyperplasia
  - dexamethasone-suppressible hyperaldosteronism
  - aldosterone producing carcinoma
* Syndrome of deoxycorticosterone excess
  - adrenal tumours
  - 11-β-hydroxylase deficiency
  - 17-α-hydroxylase deficiency
* Liddle's syndrome
* Cortisol excess
  - Cushing's disease
  - Cushing's syndrome   - adrenal tumour
                        - ectopic
                        - iatrogenic
* Oral contraceptives
* Liquorice, carbenoxolone sodium

Diagnosis

Serum potassium

Clinical suspicion of the diagnosis most often arises from a low serum potassium concentration. A diagnostic approach to the hypokalaemic hypertensive patient is depicted in Fig. 1. For serum potassium to be a reliable screening measurement, the blood sample must be obtained after the patient has been off diuretics for at least two weeks. Sodium intake should be liberal because sodium restriction can mask a tendency towards low serum potassium concentrations by reducing renal potassium excretion.

Plasma renin activity

Once the low level of serum potassium is confirmed, the diagnosis of primary aldosteronism is established by determination of PRA. Markedly suppressed PRA unresponsive to furosemide or captopril stimulation is a *sine-qua-non* for primary aldosteronism.

110

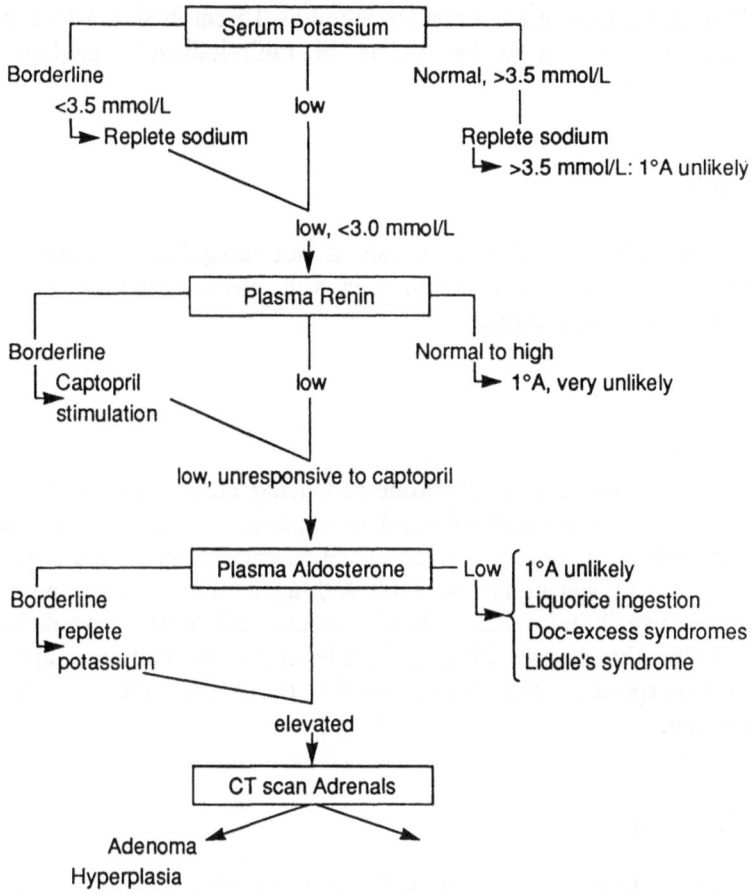

Fig. 1. Step-wise diagnostic approach to the hypokalaemic hypertensive patient

Plasma aldosterone

High aldosterone values are not essential and should be assessed in relation to the degree of hypokalaemia, which can suppress aldosterone secretion. Strikingly low levels of aldosterone in the presence of low renin suggest liquorice ingestion or corticosterone excess (tumour, enzyme deficiencies).

CT-scan

A computerized tomography (CT) scan provides definite proof of either adenoma or bilateral hyperplasia. Recent refinements in CT technology allow accurate identification of adenomas as small as 0.5 cm in size, which makes the laborious visualization by means of radio-iodinated analogues of cholesterol outdated.

Adrenal vein sampling

Occasionally, when CT-scan diagnosis is not unequivocal, adrenal vein sampling for aldosterone determination will provide definite proof for unilateral aldosterone production.

Therapy

The ultimate therapy for aldosterone-producing adrenal adenoma is uni-adrenalectomy. Patients with bilateral hyperplasia should be managed with medical treatment. It is our practice to treat all patients suspected of primary aldosteronism with spironolactone (100–400 mg/day) for at least one month. This therapy usually normalizes blood pressure and corrects hypokalaemia. Subsequently, the cases with proven adenomas are operated upon. In bilateral hyperplasia, one should go for the lowest effective dose of spironolactone.

Selected references

Hamet P (1980): Endocrine hypertension: Cushing's syndrome, acromegaly, hyperpara-thyroidism, thyrotoxicosis and hypothyroidism. In Genest J, Koiw E, Kuchel O (Eds.) *Hypertension*. McGraw-Hill, New York, pp. 964–977.

Manger WM, Gifford Jr RW (1990): Pheochromocytoma. In Laragh JH, Brenner BM (Eds.) *Hypertension: Pathophysiology, Diagnosis and Management*. Raven Press, New York, pp. 1639–1659.

Ramsey LE, Waller PC (1990): Blood pressure response to percutaneous transluminal angioplasty for renovascular hypertension: an overview of published series. *Br Med J* 300: 569–572.

Vaughan ED, Atlas S, Carey RM (1989): Hyperaldosteronism. In Vaughan ED, Carey RM (Eds.) *Adrenal Disorders*. Thieme Medical Publishers, New York, pp.243–258.

Velchik MG, Alavi A, Kressel HY, Engelman K (1989): Localization of pheochromocytoma: MIBG, CT and MRI correlation. *J Nucl Med* 30: 328–336.

Wenting GJ, Tan-Tjiong HL, Derkx FHM, De Bruyn JHB, Man in't Veld AJ, Schalekamp MAHD (1984): Split renal function after captopril in unilateral renal artery stenosis. *Br Med J* 288: 886–890.

Working Group on Renovascular Hypertension (1987): Detection, evaluation and treatment of renovascular hypertension. *Arch Intern Med* 147: 820–829.

CHAPTER 7

Non-pharmacological intervention

ROGER A. SHINTON and GARETH BEEVERS

INTRODUCTION

Few people like taking prescribed medication. In hypertension, additionally, a considerable proportion of the population have blood pressures hovering around the level at which the benefits of medication are less than spectacular. For these combined reasons, non-pharmacological interventions receive great interest from a number of patients and those looking after them.

The traditional approach to non-pharmacological management of hypertension examines a series of behavioural changes which might result in a lower pressure and the added incentive of avoiding the need for medication. An alternative approach will be adopted here. Practitioners are increasingly moving towards an approach directed at the reduction of the risk of cardiovascular disease in hypertensives. This approach can lead to the possible paradox of accepting some higher blood pressure readings on the path to a reduced cardiovascular risk.

The general principles of management are: to maintain or improve quality of life and to reduce overall morbidity and mortality. Interventions will be considered in what might be regarded as their order of importance:

REDUCING CARDIOVASCULAR RISK IN HYPERTENSIVES

Important
* Stop smoking
* Avoid overweight
* Remain physically active
* Control saturated fat intake

Probably useful
* Control alcohol intake

Possibly useful
* Reduce dietary salt
* Relaxation therapy

SMOKING CESSATION

Smoking as a cardiovascular risk factor

Those of us living in the 1990s now have the benefit of the results of numerous epidemiological investigations into the causes of heart attack and stroke. For heart attacks, it was widely argued by the 1960s that smoking (cigarettes in particular) was an important cause. All the major cohort studies indicated that current smokers had at least double the risk of a heart attack compared with non-smokers. It has more recently become apparent that strokes are also more common amongst smokers than non-smokers. This conclusion has been slower to emerge, as a minority of early studies did not observe an appreciable extra risk and also because strokes occur at an older age when the risk is less marked. The acknowledgement that cigarettes cause strokes is particularly important when considering hypertensive management as the principal benefit of lowering BP (by drugs at least) is for cerebrovascular rather than coronary diseases.

Evidence from the British Regional Heart Study, an Australian case–control study of stroke and a meta-analysis of epidemiological stroke studies have all indicated that ex-smokers are at increased risk of heart attacks and strokes. This risk may be still present up to 20 years after smoking cessation. This would suggest that smoking causes atherosclerosis itself rather than merely precipitating an acute event in vessel walls which are already diseased.

The benefit of quitting

Although many investigators have demonstrated that between 5 and 50% of patients respond to advice on smoking, the same studies have not indicated substantial gains in those who accepted advice. Both the American Multiple Risk Factor Intervention Trial and the intervention in the Whitehall cohort of civil servants yielded disappointing results. The recent data on the prolonged risk for ex-smokers may be one of the reasons explaining the observations. Few would doubt the wisdom of advising all their patients to stop smoking immediately. If the patient is young, so much the better.

Helping people to stop smoking

Some believe that doctors and others waste a lot of their time explaining the dangers of smoking. Personal experience, as well as a variety of published evidence, does suggest that people do listen and not infrequently act upon the advice proffered. Five minutes of well-focused discussion with someone in their twenties could potentially add decades to their future life and well-being.

The approach to smoking cessation by a doctor or similar worker is an individual matter. Some like to explode with wrath and others prefer the quiet and logical approach. Some physicians back up their counselling with leaflets and a host of other ploys designed to increase the impact of the message. A preferred approach should, perhaps, be that of educating the patient as fully as possible about the epidemiology and pathology of cardiovascular disease. Let the education provide the motivation.

IMPROVING COMPLIANCE WITH ADVICE TO STOP SMOKING

* Present it as the top priority
* Provide as full an explanation of the advantages as possible, mentioning perhaps:
    Atherogenesis
    Multiplication of risk factors
    Improved personal hygiene
    Other health benefits, e.g. to lungs
* Record smoking status and review as appropriate
* Provide a leaflet if available
* Remind the patient that the decision is theirs
* Advise expensive assistance (e.g. acupuncture and nicorette) as a last resort

---

AVOIDANCE OF OVERWEIGHT

The risks of overweight

There is little doubt, following analysis of several large studies, that overweight people have higher blood pressures than those who are thin. In younger people, the risk of having hypertension is several fold more likely in fat people compared with thin people. The association becomes less obvious as age advances. This is probably because, over time, other influences start to affect BP, e.g. medication, possible self-perpetuation of raised BP and myocardial and other diseases.

115

The risk of overweight for heart attack and stroke has been equivocal. Not all studies have concluded that overweight is an important independent risk factor. Most clinicians, however, strongly suspect that overweight carries substantial cardiovascular risks partly because of its association with hypertension, hyperlipidaemia and glucose intolerance. The importance of overweight may have been underestimated because smokers are often thin. Vascular damage may take decades to develop, end-stage atherosclerotics may be thin and statisticians have tended to obscure the real links of obesity by adjusting its effect for blood pressure, diabetes and hypercholesterolaemia. It does seem likely, overall, that overweight is an important cause of morbidity and mortality which is more apparent in those who are both younger and who have never smoked. When truncal obesity is considered (for example the ratio of the waist to the hip circumference) the danger seems to be more evident.

Does weight reduction lower BP?

There have now been at least 15 trials of weight reduction as a method of BP lowering. In almost all of these studies, weight reduction has been accompanied by a fall in blood pressure. The extent of the fall has varied enormously between the studies. Some suggest dramatic improvements and others rather unimpressive results. The concensus would now seem to be that weight reduction produces a useful BP reduction but that substantial falls cannot be guaranteed to the patient. The overall pattern is that, for each kilogram of weight lost, a 1 mmHg reduction of systolic or diastolic BP is achieved. An individual's BP has evolved over decades and it would be surprising if a two-month diet reversed the impact of lifelong trends. The final and most important question as to whether weight reduction prevents cardiovascular diseases and deaths has not been examined in a formal randomized trial. The University Diabetes Programme trial on diabetes, however, indicated that, for that disease, those issued with dietary advice alone had a relatively favourable outcome compared with other treatment groups. The balance of evidence would support weight loss as an important part of the successful non-pharmacological management of hypertensives and others at increased cardiovascular risk.

Achieving weight reduction

All clinicians know that compliance with advice to lose weight is poor. Many, therefore, have all but given up this approach. This is perhaps somewhat pessimistic although a large number of strategies to aid weight reduction have been explored by physicians.

Hospital clinicians perhaps get an over-pessimistic view of compliance as their clinics tend to see those with intractable problems. It does appear that a proportion of people will reduce their weight substantially when reminded of the dangers. That a few, but perhaps not all, will later regain weight has to be accepted. The doctor should educate the patient about the advantages of losing weight and thus, perhaps, provide the motivation required.

WEIGHT LOSS AND HYPERTENSION

Benefits

* Effective
* Also reduces serum cholesterol and risk of diabetes

* Also reduces other disease risks, e.g. osteoarthritis, gallstones
* Well understood and easy to monitor

Problems

* Limited compliance
* Effect less dramatic than pharmacological intervention
* May counter cultural norms
* Ideally requires action in early decades of life

A SENSIBLE APPROACH TO WEIGHT REDUCTION IN HYPERTENSIVES

* Avoid a nagging or unsympathetic approach
* Educate about the various risks of overweight
* Accept that some do have slower basal metabolism
* Insist that all can potentially reduce their weight
* Encourage appropriate physical exertion
* Monitor weight
* Use dietetic advice as appropriate
* Accept that for some it will never be a priority
* Remember: the younger the patient the more there is to gain

---

There is some evidence that dieticians providing careful assessments and recommendations improve results, as can the setting of targets and joining slimming clubs. Doctors should give some guidance about the upper limit of ideal body weight – which is around a body mass index (BMI) of 25 kg/m^2 (Table 1).

Overweight is probably better avoided than reversed. Particular attention should thus be given to young people at risk of developing hypertension or vascular diseases. An important area to concentrate on is the return to normal weight after pregnancy. Easy availability of sports facilities and a good diet are also priorities for a healthy population.

Table 1. Recommended upper limit of body weight (BMI = 25 kg/m^2)

Height			Weight		
Feet and inches		Metres	Stones and pounds		kg
4	8	1.42	7	13	50
	9	1.45	8	4	53
	10	1.47	8	7	54
	11	1.50	8	12	56
5	0	1.52	9	1	58
	1	1.55	9	6	60
	2	1.57	9	10	62
	3	1.60	10	1	64
	4	1.63	10	6	66
	5	1.65	10	10	68
	6	1.68	11	2	71
	7	1.70	11	5	72
	8	1.73	11	11	75
	9	1.75	12	1	77
	10	1.78	12	7	79
	11	1.80	12	11	81
6	0	1.83	13	2	84
	1	1.85	13	5	86
	2	1.88	13	13	88
	3	1.90	14	3	90
	4	1.93	14	9	93
	5	1.96	15	2	96

PHYSICAL EXERCISE

The risks of inactivity

The risks of inactivity in the causation of hypertension have not been easy to study in an entirely satisfactory manner. The principal problem is the difficulty in making suitable measurements of a persons activity levels. Paffenbarger, however, demonstrated that university students who did not participate in university sports were more likely to develop hypertension in later years. Measures of increased physical fitness also seem to correlate with lower BPs.

Many large epidemiological studies have examined the role of exercise in the development of coronary heart disease and most have concluded that a beneficial effect exists. The balance of evidence also suggests exercise protects against strokes. The amount of exercise required to reduce cardiovascular risk is not clear. It is highly likely that the greater the energy expended, the greater the reduction in cardiovascular risk. Almost all study results would be consistent with this concept. The risks of vigorous exercise for cardiovascular disease have probably been overstated.

Exercise for hypertensives

There have now been a series of randomized studies assessing the hypotensive effect of physical activity. The results of these do suggest a small but useful reduction in blood pressure. It is now more widely accepted that the whole population and hypertensives in particular, should be encouraged to partake in regular and preferably kinetic (rather than static) physical activity. As well as probably lowering blood pressure, it reduces serum cholesterol, weight and overall cardiovascular risk.

In encouraging this increase in exercise, a hurdle of anxiety about the risks of exercise has to be overcome. Doctors and their patients know that while partaking in sports, BP rises, often to a considerable degree. This is then seen as a risk which can usefully be avoided. Activities, however, which temporarily raise BP may, paradoxically, lower baseline 'clinic' or 'home' BP and thus overall cardiovascular risk. To reflect this anxiety, a variety of sports require hypertensives to produce medical certificates before being allowed to partake. This barrier is most unfortunate for otherwise fit hypertensive people.

The concerns over activity and cardiovascular disease are based on collected case series whose heart attack occurred during vigorous sports –

119

notably squash. There is currently a lack of epidemiologically satisfactory evidence that such cases have arisen other than by coincidence. Legitimate concern does, however, still remain. This is particularly so with isometric rather than dynamic exercise.

An approach which can accommodate the worries and the potential gains is that of gradually increased levels of activity. This is now adopted post-myocardial infarction with very acceptable results. There are several practical problems in encouraging hypertensives to exercise. A principal problem is that the habit of exercising has frequently not developed. Sporting and social activities tend to go hand in hand, so social inhibitions, which are easy to comprehend, will deter many. Also, sporting facilities in many countries are far more accessible to those with higher incomes.

EXERCISE IN HYPERTENSIVES

Problems	Suggestions
* Few have exercised recently	* Build up activity levels very gradually
* A proportion are restricted by angina, peripheral vascular disease, osteoarthritis, etc.	* Point out the benefits of exercise for these conditions
* Opportunities for exercise may be restricted	* Suggest time is put aside as it is important
	* Encourage a sport or activity which might be enjoyed

Further problems arise in hypertensives because of the frequent association with diseases which limit physical activity, for example angina, intermittent claudication, cerebrovascular disease, osteoarthritis of the knee and gout. For these patients, the limitations are not easily overcome and have to be accepted. It is reassuring, however, that for the majority of these conditions the benefits of exercise have been clearly demonstrated. It has now been shown that heart failure, too, may benefit from an appropriate increase in exercise.

DIETARY FAT AND BLOOD PRESSURE

Dietary fat and cardiovascular disease

Controversy continues to rage over the importance of dietary fat in cardiovascular disease. While there is general agreement that cardiovascular event rates rise with serum cholesterol levels, not all accept that lowering dietary saturated fat brings about substantial overall health benefits. A majority of physicians would, however, now accept the need to discourage diets rich in saturated fats. This advice applies to the whole population but particularly to those at higher cardiovascular risk. It now seems that the risks of excessive saturated fats apply to cerebrovascular thrombosis as well as coronary heart disease. There remains a possibility, however, that cerebral haemorrhage is positively associated with a low serum (and thus probably also dietary) cholesterol. As cerebral haemorrhage is a relatively rare form of stroke, it does not affect the overall conclusions on dietary advice.

Dietary fat and hypertension

There has been considerable interest in the observation that vegetarians have substantially lower blood pressures than meat eaters. Although the reason for this may be their low saturated fat intake, variables such as lower levels of obesity and more exercise may explain some of the findings. There have now been over 10 trials examining the possible hypotension effects of various dietary fat modifications. A switch to a vegetarian or reduced saturated-fat diet may slightly lower BP but the trials have only lasted for a matter of weeks or months. Whether substantial falls in BP could be obtained by a long-term vegetarian diet is currently unclear.

The addition of oily fish to the diet has been claimed to have both hypotensive and other beneficial cardiovascular effects. This area is promising but, again, remains somewhat inconclusive at present.

Although reducing saturated fat intake can often usefully be recommended to hypertensives, it would be misleading to predict major reductions in blood pressure. The principal benefit would arise from a reduction of the overall cardiovascular risk. Avoidance of overweight and encouragement of physical activities can be stressed as benefiting both blood pressure and cholesterol levels.

There is an increasing trend to measurement of serum cholesterol and its subfractions in people presenting with hypertension. Although this form of screening cannot be regarded as essential, it does help the physicians to concentrate dietary advice on those individuals with particularly high levels. A majority of hypertensives do seem to have cholesterol levels well above the ideal value (5.2 mmol/L).

Dietary advice, preferably from a dietician, should be available for those requesting more specific guidance on improving the balance of fats in their diet. An increase in the polyunsaturated-to-saturated fat ratio may well be sensible but questions remain about the value of eating more polyunsaturated fat.

ALCOHOL

Alcohol and blood pressure

A variety of epidemiological and clinical studies now point to alcohol as an agent which elevates blood pressure. The epidemiological evidence from the Kaiser Permanente Study suggests that light alcohol drinking is associated with lower blood pressures than average but heavy alcohol consumption causes blood pressure elevation. The hypertensive effect of heavy drinking appears to exist with all forms of alcohol, i.e. beer, wine, spirits and fortified wines.

It is now considered quite possible that the pressor effects of alcohol are short lived. Alcohol may, therefore, cause 'pseudohypertension' rather than 'real' hypertension. This uncertainty means that the risks or benefits of alcohol on cardiovascular disease requires study of important disease endpoints such as heart attack or stroke. Case-control studies on the risks of alcohol for stroke have usually but not always indicated that heavy drinking carries an increased risk. Light drinking is associated with a reduced risk but the association may not be causal. In a cohort of American nurses, alcohol (taken mainly in moderation) seemed to confer an overall protective effect on stroke. Other cohorts have found little effect.

Cohort studies have examined the risks of heavy drinking for coronary heart disease and, in general, not found any striking relationships from which firm conclusions can be drawn. For these reasons stringent advice about precise levels of recommended alcohol consumption to avoid cardiovascular disease is premature. Clearly alcohol remains hazardous for a wide range of other serious medical and social problems.

Advice to cut back on alcohol consumption

Few clinicians would disagree that cardiovascular and/or other health benefits can be achieved by restricting alcohol consumption to less than 30 units* per week and probably less in women. A hypertensive patient would surely be pleased to see a reduction in his blood pressure brought about by a degree of abstinence. Much alcohol in Northern Europe is consumed as beer. Beer drinking has been shown to be associated with increased overweight. Moderation in this instance should also mean control of weight is made easier.

What is the evidence that people modify their drinking habits after appropriate advice? A small randomized study conducted in Birmingham indicated an appreciable drop in blood markers for alcohol (γ-glutamyl transferase) in those advised to restrict their alcohol intake. A small but non-significant fall in blood pressure was also seen. Experience tells most doctors that enough people do accept their advice to make the effort worthwhile.

ALCOHOL ADVICE IN HYPERTENSIVE PATIENTS

* Patients frequently appear to act upon advice.
* Regular heavy drinking should be discouraged for other medical and social reasons as well as for possible cardiovascular benefits.
* Excessive calories in beer/lager may be an additional hazard.
* The definition of excessive drinking is debated and varies from 14 to 71 drinks or units* per week; 30 units seems a sensible compromise. It should perhaps be lower in women.
* The red blood cell mean corpuscular volume and γ-glutamyl transferase are useful but not as reliable as the patient's word.

SALT

Whether or not salt has an important role in causing cardiovascular disease remains unresolved. The world-wide 'Intersalt' project has not shown salt to be an important cause of hypertension across all the populations studied. The

---

* 1 unit = 8–10 g alcohol = ½ pint of beer, 1 tot of spirit, or 1 glass of wine, sherry or port.

very small blood pressure rise with age, however, seen in the primitive, low-salt eating populations remains intriguing. The salt story will continue to run.

Intervention trials of low-salt diets to lower blood pressures have shown some success. The pattern, however, has not been uniform and at present it remains possible rather than probable that a reduction in dietary salt will affect health. It is possible that in groups such as non-insulin dependent diabetics a more pronounced response will be seen.

A reduction in dietary sodium to 80–100 mmol (about 5 g of salt) per day can be achieved without making the diet unpalatable to Westernized communities.

It would be premature to suggest that all hypertensives should be advised to reduce their salt intake. Clinicians may like to suggest the possibility of a benefit to those patients who inquire or in those who want to try any non-pharmacological hypotensive approach which might bear fruit.

Potassium as well as sodium intake has been assessed in association with hypertension. There is some evidence that a high output of potassium (a likely marker of high dietary input) is associated with lower blood pressure. Not surprisingly, therefore, the urinary sodium/potassium ratio has also been investigated. At present conclusions have to be limited but advice to eat plenty of vegetables which have a high potassium/low sodium content would seen sensible on many counts. Taking potassium supplements has been shown to be of no obvious benefit in lowering blood pressure.

STRESS

Much importance has been ascribed to stress in the development of cardiovascular disease. Many people do believe it is a cardinal precipitant of heart attacks, strokes and high blood pressure. Examination of the research literature, however, fails to find substantive support for the stress hypothesis. The principal problem, of course, is the inadequacy of any definition of 'stress'. What is more plausible is that individuals under pressure tend to lead life styles more conducive to the development of cardiovascular disease. Certainly, low social class is strongly linked to an increased risk of all cardiovascular diseases. It may be that part of this is related to education but this is unlikely to be the whole story.

Trials of relaxation therapy have yielded some improvement in blood pressure levels. Whether this effect is clinically important has not yet been established.

MULTIPLE RISK FACTOR INTERVENTION

The preceding paragraphs are clearly not alternative strategies but are often complementary. Most would agree that advice on all the important life-style factors should be given to both hypertensives and non-hypertensives when the opportunity arises. A randomized trial of this non-pharmacological approach has, however, never been conducted with the endpoints of heart attack and stroke. Circumstantial evidence supporting this approach comes from, amongst others, Chicago where substantial blood pressure falls were seen in those who had modified a range of adverse risk factors for hypertension. It would now be difficult to conduct an appropriate trial as many would consider it both unethical and impractical to withhold appropriate advice on life-style related risk factors.

Large-scale multiple risk factor intervention trials, involving pharmacological and non-pharmacological approaches, have taken place in Europe and America over the past two decades. The results, disappointingly, did not show appreciable differences between the intervention and control groups. The principal observation, however, was a substantial decline in cardiovascular morbidity and mortality in all those studied. The message seemed to get through to all the participants!

Only a minority of those in medical practice now feel sceptical about the positive benefits of educating patients and communities on health-promoting life styles. Few would also argue that political and taxation policies can help enhance the adoption of safer personal habits. It is likely that improved education will eventually lead to subsequent political developments in the search for improved cardiovascular health.

FAILURE OF THE NON-PHARMACOLOGICAL APPROACH

Not all those hoping for BP control by non-pharmacological methods will be successful. Some patients will modify their life styles yet still have a BP which would probably benefit from being lowered with the aid of drugs. In others the modifications of habit will not be achieved for a variety of complex personal and social reasons. Physicians must accept the failures with the successes and maintain a constructive and sympathetic approach. Current evidence suggests that if the diastolic BP remains persistently over 100 mmHg, despite several months of non-pharmacological management, drug treatment should be instituted.

Selected references

Cook DG, Shaper AG, Pocock SJ, Kussick SJ (1986): Giving up smoking and the risk of heart attacks. *Lancet* 2: 1376–1380.

Donnan GA, Adena MA, O'Malley HM, McNeill JJ, Doyle AE, Neill GC (1989): Smoking as a risk factor for cerebral ischaemia. *Lancet* 2: 643–647.

Intersalt Co-operative Research Group (1988): Intersalt: an international study of electrolyte excretion and blood pressure. Results for 24 hour urinary sodium and potassium excretion. *Br Med J* 297: 319–328.

Kannel WB, Brand N, Skinner JJ, Dawker TR, McNamara PM (1967): The relation of adiposity to blood pressure and development of hypertension. The Framingham Study. *Ann Int Med* 67: 48–59.

Klatsky AL, Friedman GD, Siegelamh AB, Gerard MJ (1977): Alcohol consumption among white, black or oriental men and women: Kaiser-Permanente multiphasic health examination data. *Am J Epidemiol* 105: 311–323.

Maheswaran R, Beevers M, Beevers DG (1988): Evaluation of alcohol advice in hypertensive patients. *J Hypertension* 6: 946.

Nelson L, Jennings GL, Elser MD, Korner PI (1986): Effects of changing levels of physical activity on blood pressure and haemodynamics in essential hypertension. *Lancet* 2: 473–476.

Paffenbarger RS, Thorne MC, Wing AL (1968): Chronic disease in former college students VIII. Characteristics in youth predisposing to hypertension in later life. *Am J Epidemiol* 88: 25–32.

Patel C, Marmot MG, Terry DJ, Carruthers M, Hunt B, Patel M (1985): Trial of relaxation in reducing coronary risk: four year follow up. *Br Med J* 290: 1103–1106.

Potter JF, Beevers DG (1984): Pressor effect of alcohol in hypertension. *Lancet* 1: 119–122.

Rose G, Hamilton PJS (1978): A randomised controlled trial of the effect on middle-aged men of advice to stop smoking. *J Epidemiol Comm Health* 32: 275–281.

Shinton RA, Beevers DG (1989): Meta-analysis of the relation between cigarette smoking and stroke. *Br Med J* 298: 789–794.

Shinton RA, Dodson PM, Beevers DG (1989): Hypertension and dietary fat. *J Human Hypertension* 3: 73–78.

Staessen J, Fagard R, Amery A (1988): The relationship between body weight and blood pressure. *J Human Hypertension* 2: 207–217.

Stampfer MJ, Colditz GA, Willett WC, Speizer FE, Hennekens CH (1988): A prospective study of moderate alcohol consumption and the risk of coronary disease and stroke in women. *N Engl J Med* 319: 267–273.

Welin L, Svardsudd K, Wilhelmsen L, Larsson B, Tibblin G (1987): Analysis of risk factors for stroke in a cohort of men born in 1913. *N Engl J Med* 317: 521–526.

CHAPTER 8

Drug treatment: efficacy and adverse effects. Specific responses in patient sub-groups and treatment approach

GASTONE LEONETTI and CESARE CUSPIDI

Introduction

Once the diagnosis of hypertension has been established and the initial evaluation completed, the clinician must decide whether to initiate non-pharmacological and/or pharmacological treatment and in the latter case how to choose from the vast array of agents now available. Treatment of patients with hypertension has attained a remarkable state of sophistication.

The thiazide diuretics and more recently the β-blockers have been the traditional first-step agents in the stepped-care approach to therapy of hypertension. Stepped-care therapy was not intended to be a rigid algorithm that had to be followed in all cases, but rather it was intended to be a set of guidelines for treatment based on experience and arrived at by consensus. When the first stepped-care proposal (Fig. 1) was introduced, the only options other than diuretics for initial therapy were methyldopa, reserpine, guanethidine or hydralazine, and the diuretic agents were by far preferable to any of the other drugs or they had to be combined with the latter anyway to prevent or correct 'pseudotolerance' due to water and sodium retention. In 1978 the WHO (Fig. 2) and later in 1984 the third Joint National Committee on Detection, Evaluation and Treatment of High Blood Pressure (JNC) suggested an alternative as first step: either a thiazide diuretic agent or a β-blocker both at less than full dose. More recently the WHO and the fourth JNC reports recommended alternatives for step one, including calcium antagonists, angiotensin converting enzyme (ACE) inhibitors or α_1-adrenergic receptor inhibitors. A proposal to liberalize stepped care even further will be discussed at the end of this chapter.

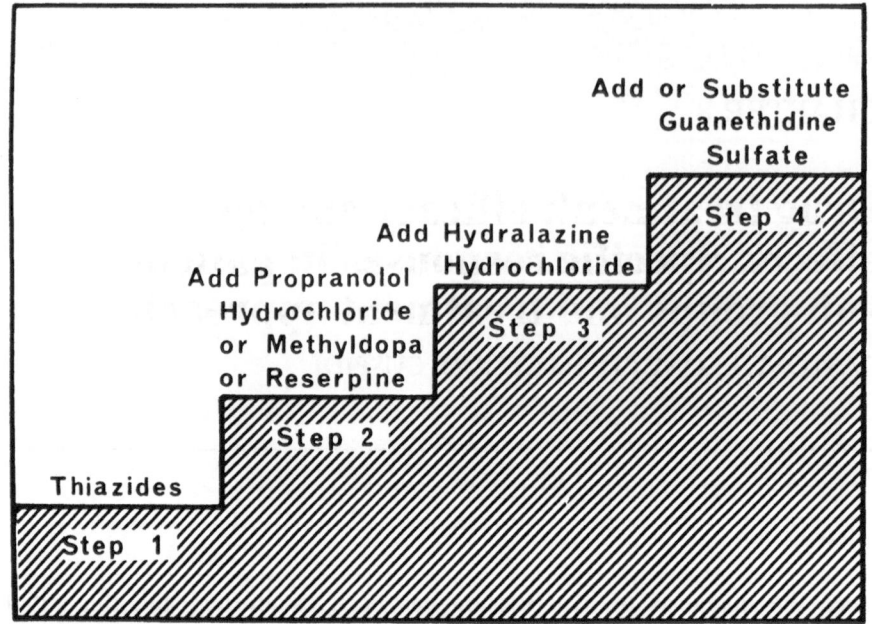

Fig. 1 Stepped-care antihypertensive program suggested by the US Joint National Committee on Detection, Evaluation and Treatment of High Blood Pressure (1977)

THE POTENTIAL OF ANTIHYPERTENSIVE DRUGS

If hypertensive patients do not respond to non-pharmacological treatment they will obviously require drug therapy. The decision which drug to choose for first-line therapy depends on many reasons: efficacy, side-effects, associated diseases, dosage schedule, demography, cost, mechanism of drug action and individual aspects of pathophysiology. Selection of the antihypertensive drug for the individual must be based on the sum of the available knowledge, derived both from pharmacological studies and from epidemiological and empirical experience. On the following pages, the merits and potential disadvantages of the different classes of current antihypertensives will be discussed in the following sequence: diuretics, β-blockers, calcium antagonists, ACE inhibitors, α-blockers and the single available serotonin$_2$ blocker.

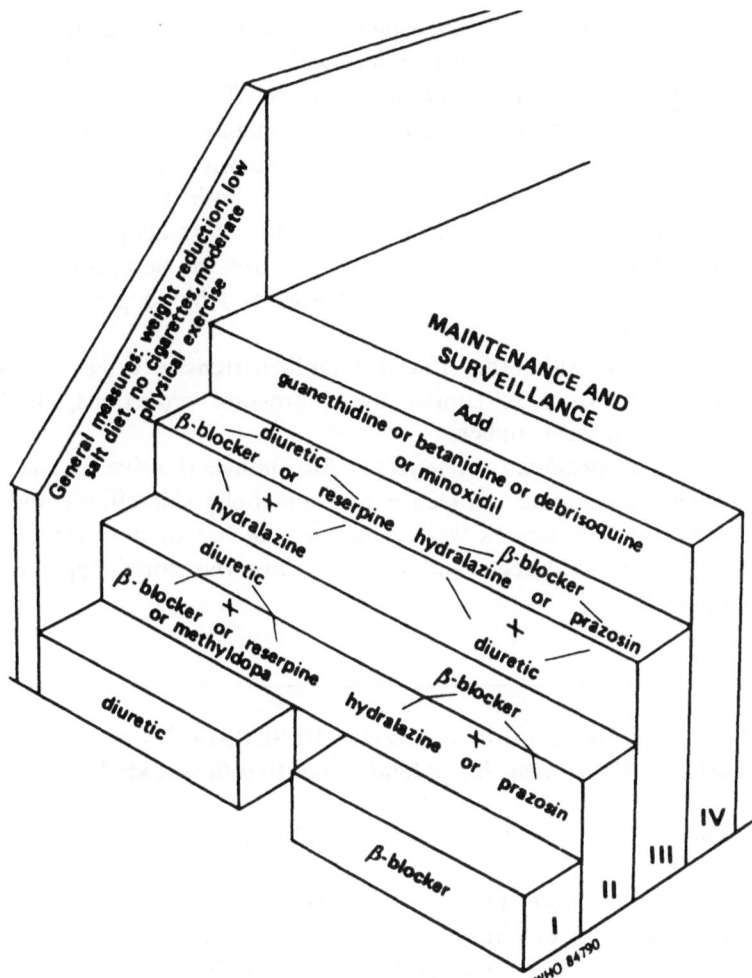

Fig. 2 Stepped-care antihypertensive programme suggested by the WHO Expert Committee (1978)

Diuretics

The thiazide diuretics were introduced into medicine in 1958 after the discovery of chlorothiazide and were originally indicated for the treatment of other diseases (i.e. sodium and water retention secondary to cardiac failure, renal insufficiency, etc.) but their most extensive use has turned out to be the treatment of hypertensive subjects. The original use of diuretics in patients with oedema, where an obvious dose–response curve of the natriuretic and

129

diuretic effects was present, can explain the initial use of high doses of diuretics in the treatment of hypertension, without there being any evidence of a dose–response curve of their antihypertensive efficacy.

Efficacy. Clinical experience with diuretics (mainly those of the thiazide type) has been very extensive. It has been shown that diuretics cause statistically and clinically significant reductions both in systolic (10–12 mmHg) and diastolic (6–8n mmHg) blood pressure. If we adopt 90 mmHg as the value indicating normalization of blood pressure, the percentage of mild or moderate hypertensive patients with normalized blood pressure varies between 40 and 70%.

When compared with other first-line antihypertensive drugs, diuretics have been shown to cause similar blood pressure reductions, both in short-term and long-term studies.

Subjective and metabolic side-effects. All antihypertensive agents have both tolerable and serious subjective and metabolic side-effects and this clearly applies to thiazides as well. The clinician has to be aware of the incidence of such side-effects and to judge how this could apply to the individual patient.

INCIDENCE OF THE MOST COMMON SIDE-EFFECTS FROM THIAZIDES (among 425 patients from 10 different studies)*

>3%	1 – 3%	<1%
Headache	Vertigo	Hyponatraemia
Tiredness	Palpitations	Depression
Weakness	Light headedness	Loss of libido
	Nausea	Hypotension
	Rush	Chest pain
		Visual disturbances

* Modified from McMahon. Management of Essential Hypertension. Futura Publishing Company Inc. 1978, 35

Taking into account that diuretics were proposed by the JNC and WHO as first-step drugs because they tend to be well-tolerated, it was rather surprising to learn from the Medical Research Council Trial that the incidence of withdrawals for side-effects was no less than 17.1% in men and

12.8% in women treated with diuretics. The most frequent subjective side-effects were sexual dysfunction (22.6% vs 10.1% with placebo, $p < 0.05$) exertional dyspnoea, muscle pain in men, and dry mouth (28.1 vs 13.6% with placebo, $p < 0.05$), exertional dyspnoea, paraesthesia and blocked nose in women.

Thiazides have been shown to increase plasma lipid levels, to reduce glucose tolerance and lower plasma potassium and magnesium: these metabolic changes can persist beyond the first few months of therapy (although there is some controversy about lipids). The Hypertension Detection and Follow-up Study and the Medical Research Council Trial have shown that the metabolic changes and the plasma potassium reduction are still present after years of diuretic therapy, when compared with the placebo group. It is important to note however that the diuretic doses employed in these trials were higher than current low-dosage levels which have a similar antihypertensive efficacy and a minor interference on plasma potassium and glucose tolerance.

Comorbidity. The presence of concomitant disease, which can be helped or worsened by antihypertensive treatment, should be a major factor in the choice of the initial therapy for hypertension.

Hypertensive patients with gout or elevated levels of uric acid should not be treated with diuretics because they decrease the renal excretion of uric acid and therefore raise plasma concentrations. Similarly, patients with hypercholesterolaemia may not qualify for treatment with diuretics.

By contrast, patients with congestive heart failure due to systolic dysfunction are of course well off when receiving diuretics. In patients with chronic renal failure, diastolic blood pressure tends to be positively correlated with plasma volume, and effective diuretic agents (i.e. loop diuretics) should therefore be the first type of agent to be used here. Obese patients have some expansion of total body fluid volumes and this may justify the use of thiazides as first choice. Diuretics of the thiazide type reduce renal excretion of calcium and therefore can be used in hypertensive patients with hypercalciuria, calcium oxalate nephrolithiasis or chronic calcium deficit.

Diabetic patients are an important and worrying subgroup of hypertensive patients. Diuretic drugs are known to produce insulin resistance and to worsen glucose tolerance, although this effect is less when total body potassium is maintained. Other antihypertensive agents, being neutral with respect to glucose tolerance, are of course preferable to thiazides.

Dosage schedule and cost. Since all classes of antihypertensives are currently available in formulations suitable for once-a-day or twice-a-day therapy, the simple dosage schedule of thiazides and the favourable effect on compliance is no longer an argument in favour of the latter.

Although the cost of drugs may not be a principal matter, its impact cannot be disregarded; quite a number of patients have to pay for their own medication. In this regard it should be stressed that thiazides are by far the cheapest antihypertensives available for normotherapy. Even the combination with a potassium-sparing agent (triamterene or amiloride) has only a modest effect on price.

β-Adrenergic-receptor blocking agents

The β-adrenergic-receptor blocking agents were introduced in 1965 and like diuretics were originally intended for the treatment of another disease (angina pectoris). Their use was soon extended to the treatment of hypertension as initiated by Prichard.

Efficacy. β-Blockers are effective antihypertensive agents and cause significant blood pressure reductions over placebo treatment.

Adequate comparative data on the use of thiazide diuretic agents and β-blockers as monotherapy have been provided by several long-term trials and many short-term ones. On balance β-blockers have been shown to be equipotent to diuretics as well as calcium-antagonists and ACE inhibitors: some variations in different studies may be due to preselection of study populations.

Subjective and metabolic side-effects. β-Blockers, like diuretics, have been advocated as first-choice drugs for the treatment of hypertension because they produce few symptomatic side-effects. In the mean time, however, the Medical Research Council Trial has shown that in their propranolol-treated group 15.5% of the men and 18% of the women had to be withdrawn mainly because of side-effects. The more frequent side-effects were exertional dyspnoea (27.9% vs 16.4% with placebo, $p < 0.05$), blocked nose, slowed walking pace and paraesthesias in men and women, and cold or numb digits (29.3% vs 15.6% with placebo, $p < 0.05$), particularly in women. In addition it has been shown in several trials that β-blockers may cause significant increases in the concentration of serum triglycerides and decreases in cardioprotective high-density lipoprotein cholesterol; these effects are blunted or absent in β-blockers with substantial intrinsic sympathomimetic activity or vasodilatory properties.

Comorbidity. β-Blockers deserve particular attention with regard to concomitant diseases because their administration may either be useful or harmful depending on the background of history and physical examination.

Patients with a history of chronic obstructive airway disease or congestive heart failure ought not to be treated with β-blockers, because the symptoms of concomitant diseases are apt to worsen during treatment. Sick sinus syndrome, peripheral vascular disease and Raynaud's phenomenon are also prohibitive. Such contraindications to the use of β-blockers are due to the inhibition of both β_1- and β_2-receptor-mediated effects; they can therefore not be avoided by using β_1-selective blockers, particularly when high doses are given.

By contrast, patients with coronary heart disease can improve with β-blockers through a decrease in cardiac work and oxygen demand. Patients with hyperthyroidism or excessive anxiety may experience severe palpitations, which can be controlled with β-blockers.

Dosage schedule and cost. Currently available β-blockers can be administered once-a-day or twice-a-day as has been shown by 24 hour blood pressure monitoring.

The cost of β-blockers is higher than that of diuretics, though still way below the price of the newer antihypertensive agents.

Mechanism of drug action and 'individual pathophysiology' of hypertension. Most β-blockers reduce blood pressure by reducing cardiac output and by leaving total peripheral resistance unchanged, thus theoretically making them ideal for the treatment of young hypertensive individuals with hyperkinetic circulation, characterized by increased cardiac output. In practice, however, middle-of-the-road hypertension with normal or even reduced cardiac output, normal heart rates and increased total peripheral vascular resistance tend to respond equally well to β-blockade as the selective category of young hypertensives referred to above.

In the same vein, β-blockers were once thought to be particularly effective in patients with 'renin-dependent' hypertension; this was based on the assumption that the primary mechanism of drug action was their ability to block a hyperactive renin–angiotensin–aldosterone system. However, it has since become clear that patients without overt renin dependency also respond quite well to β-blockade. This suggests that either our interpretation of pathophysiological sequelae or our expertise with respect to the antihypertensive mechanisms of β-blockade remains to be perfected.

Calcium antagonists

Calcium has become recognized as one of the important ions controlling a variety of functions. A potential role of calcium in hypertension has been suggested with respect to sympathetic neurotransmission, release of norepinephrine from nerve terminals, renal release of renin, aldosterone secretion, vascular smooth muscle tone, and responsiveness to adrenoceptor agonists. Thus, it is hardly surprising that drugs inhibiting the cellular influx of calcium have proved to be interesting antihypertensive agents.

From a clinical point of view, all calcium antagonists share one haemodynamic mechanism in that they reduce total peripheral vascular resistance. This class of drugs has been variously named: calcium antagonists, calcium-channel blockers and calcium-entry blockers. In Europe the term calcium antagonists has gained preference. Chemically the calcium antagonists can be subdivided into three groups: dihydropyridines (e.g. nifedipine), diphenylalkylamines (e.g. verapamil) and benzothiazepines (e.g. diltiazem). Calcium antagonists inhibit calcium entry into vascular and cardiac muscle cells, blocking the potential-operated channels, that is through the channels activated by a change in membrane potential; although an interference with receptor-operated channels activated by norepinephrine may also contribute to their effect. At the cardiac level, the calcium antagonists can modify the contractile behaviour of myocardial cells, as well as the automaticity of sino-atrial and atrioventricular nodes and tracts.

The differences in chemical structure between the three groups and their respective tissue affinities are probably responsible for the different effects of verapamil, nifedipine and diltiazem at cardiac and vascular levels respectively. Thus, in man, verapamil exhibits the strongest chronotropic and inotropic depressant actions, which are absent in nifedipine. The effects of diltiazem are intermediate. On the other hand, the dihydropyridine derivatives are the most potent vasodilators of the three and this degree of vasodilatation tends to be accompanied by reflex tachycardia.

Efficacy. The antihypertensive efficacy of calcium antagonists in mild to moderate hypertension has been reported both in short- and long-term studies.

Verapamil has been shown to be more potent than placebo, the percentage of patients achieving a diastolic blood pressure of less than 90 mmHg varying from 31 to 92% in three different studies. From intra-arterial pressure monitoring studies over 24 hours, the mean daytime blood pressure change was −22/−16 mmHg, without obvious changes in circadian rhythm. On the average, verapamil has been shown to be equipotent to diuretics and β-blockers. Similar findings have been reported on diltiazem and nifedipine. Nifedipine was found to be equipotent to β-blockers, diuretics and ACE inhibitors.

Unfortunately, there is little information about the comparative effectiveness of the different categories of calcium antagonists. Although clinical experience suggests little differences in antihypertensive actions, controlled trials addressing their comparative therapeutic value should be carried out for further assessment. Another more important uncertainty with regard to all 3 categories is how long-term blood pressure control with calcium antagonists would compare with the earlier drugs in preventing the cardiovascular complications of hypertension.

Comorbidity. Concomitant diseases, as coronary insufficiency and congestive heart failure can improve with the administration of calcium antagonists and therefore may present specific indications for their use in hypertensive patients; some caution should be exercised though with regard to verapamil in patients with congestive heart failure. Calcium antagonists do not appear to be contraindicated in patients with diabetes mellitus, chronic obstructive airway disease or increased levels of lipoproteins. Hypertensive patients with peripheral vascular disease, left ventricle hypertrophy or renal insufficiency can have their blood pressure lowered with calcium antagonists without deterioration or even with an improvement of concomitant disease.

Patients with migraine ought not to be treated with calcium antagonists, in particular those of the dihydropyridine group, despite some claims to the contrary.

Particular attention should be paid to the association of β-blockers and verapamil in patients with a history of congestive heart failure. On the other hand, verapamil is extremely useful in patients with proxysmal artrial tachycardia.

Subjective and metabolic side-effects. Calcium antagonists have a varying propensity for producing unwanted effects and many of them are the results of the pharmacodynamic properties of these agents (Table 1). Diltiazem seems to produce the fewest adverse reactions of the available calcium antagonists. With slow-release formulations of verapamil and nifedipine the incidence and severity of many side-effects is significantly reduced.

Table 1. Incidence (%) of most common categories of adverse events in patients receiving nifedipine or verapamil slow-release

	Nifedipine (%)	Verapamil (%)
Headache	7.2	1.9
Flushing	5.3	0.1
Dizziness	3.1	3.5
Gastrointestinal symptoms	5.2	2.7
Ankle oedema	2.1	1.5
Bradycardia	0	1.3
Constipation	2.3	8.1

Calcium antagonists do not cause metabolic side-effects and are well tolerated, e.g. by diabetic patients, although some interference of calcium antagonists on insulin release at pancreatic level and on insulin action at cellular level has been suggested.

Dosage schedule and cost. The first pharmaceutical formulations of nifedipine, verapamil and diltiazem had the disadvantage of a short duration of action; in the mean time this problem has been solved by the advent of new calcium antagonists and new pharmaceutical formulations allowing a once-a-day or twice-a-day administration with adequate 24-hour blood pressure control.

The cost of calcium antagonists is much higher than that of thiazide diuretics and higher than that of β-blockers.

Mechanism of drug action and pathophysiology of hypertension. Blood pressure elevation is usually based on increased total peripheral vascular resistance. From a pathophysiological point of view, therefore, calcium antagonists, by causing a reduction in total peripheral vascular resistance without a clinically relevant negative inotropic action, should represent an optimal drug. Furthermore, in contrast to previously available direct vasodilators, calcium antagonists do not cause sodium and water retention or a lasting activation of sympathetic nervous system activity.

Angiotensin converting enzyme inhibitors (ACE inhibitors)

The introduction of angiotensin converting enzyme inhibitors has permitted a reassessment of antihypertensive therapy at the initial and subsequent steps. ACE inhibitors were developed after the elucidation of the importance of the renin–angiotensin–aldosterone system in the pathophysiology of hypertension. Furthermore, the introduction of these agents has permitted an advance in adjusting therapy to the individual patients.

Efficacy. The ACE inhibitors were introduced initially for the treatment of angiotensin-dependent forms of hypertension (e.g. due to renal artery stenosis) and for patients with severe hypertension refractory to other forms of antihypertensive therapy. Furthermore, the first available ACE inhibitor, captopril, was used for the treatment of severely hypertensive patients with collagen vascular disease who usually had renal parenchymal functional involvement. In these patients, high doses were used initially. This has led to a high incidence of adverse effects (below).

Later these drugs were found to be effective at low dosages in ordinary patients with uncomplicated hypertension, regardless of their renin status. When compared with diuretics, β-blockers and calcium antagonists, ACE inhibitors cause similar blood pressure reductions, the percentage of patients attaining diastolic blood pressures below 90 mmHg ranging from 40 to 70%.

Although there is a paucity of data on the relative effectiveness of different ACE inhibitors (captopril, enalapril, lisinopril etc.), clinical experience suggests little difference.

136

Comorbidity. The ACE inhibitors are particularly beneficial in hypertensive patients with congestive heart failure, since both reduction in blood pressure, mediated by a decrease in peripheral vascular resistance, and improvement in venous compliance unload the heart. ACE inhibitors are also effective in reducing left ventricular hypertrophy as well as improving diastolic function. The drugs lack any negative interferences with lipoprotein and glucose metabolism. It has further been shown that they can delay the deterioration of glomerular filtration in diabetic patients with nephropathy and proteinuria. In patients with renal failure, ACE inhibitors must be employed at lower doses if only because most of them are excreted with urine in the active form; with this precaution drug accumulation can be avoided.

Although ACE inhibitors are effective in reducing blood pressure in patients with renovascular hypertension, their use in this setting may be counterproductive in that they abolish compensatory AII-dependent efferent arteriolar constriction and therefore may cause a dramatic drop in glomerular filtration pressure and rate.

Metabolic and subjective side-effects. Proteinuria and neutropenia caused major concern in the past, when captopril was administered in high doses and/or in patients with advanced renal failure secondary to collagen or autoimmune disease. After ACE inhibitors became employed at lower doses, in patients with uncomplicated mild and moderate hypertension, the frequency of neutropenia and/or proteinuria rapidly declined.

Less severe side-effects include rash (6%), taste disturbance (3.1%), headache (5.6%) and lassitude/fatigue (2.5%): all of these effects disappear on withdrawal of the drug or even by decreasing the dose. An important adverse effect is a disturbing cough that disappears upon withdrawal of the medication. This cough was not originally recognised as a side-effect because it used to be ascribed to intercurrent disorders: this explains the different incidences reported. An increased level of kinins at the pulmonary level, resulting from converting enzyme inhibition, has been suggested as a possible mechanism. A rare, but potentially dangerous side-effect is angioneurotic oedema. Although all of these side-effects may occur with any of the available ACE inhibitors, rash and taste disturbance tend to be more frequently observed with captopril, and headache and fatigue with enalapril. There has been no clinically relevant effect on serum potassium levels unless supplemental potassium or potassium-retaining agents are concomitantly administered: under these circumstances hyperkalaemia may occur.

Dosage schedule and cost. Although initially captopril was given three times a day, later studies have shown that 25 or 50 mg twice a day is as effective. More recently it has been shown that a single oral dose of 100 mg of captopril can produce a 24-hour blood pressure reduction. Enalapril and lisinopril appear to be effective during once-a-day administration.

The cost of angiotensin converting enzyme inhibitors is one of the highest of all antihypertensives.

Mechanism of drug action and pathophysiology of hypertension. Like calcium antagonists, ACE inhibitors are vasodilating agents and lower blood pressure by reducing total peripheral vascular resistance. The mechanism underlying the vasodilatation is complex and not fully understood: while the acute antihypertensive effect is proportionally correlated to the levels of circulating plasma renin this correlation no longer exists during long-term treatment. In addition to the alternative hypotheses proposed to explain the long-term antihypertensive effect (inhibition of bradykinin degradation, interference with catecholamine release and reuptake, baroreceptor resetting), it has been recently suggested that inhibition of the tissue renin–angiotensin system may play a crucial role. The inhibition of this autocrine/paracrine system could also explain the absence of reflex tachycardia and sodium and water retention, as well as the non-mechanical component of the regression of left ventricle hypertrophy.

OTHER CLASSES OF ANTIHYPERTENSIVE DRUGS

α_1-Adrenergic blockers

Prazosin, the first selective α_1 inhibitor, was introduced for the treatment of arterial hypertension in 1976 and was obviously preferable to non-selective α-blockers because it appeared to maintain the local receptor–operator control system, thus preventing tachycardia and pseudotolerance. Terazosin and doxazosin have a rather similar chemical structure, but unlike prazosin they can be used once a day.

Selective α_1-inhibitors lower blood pressure effectively by reducing vascular tone in the resistance and capacitance vessels. Prazosin and doxazosin have been found to be equipotent in lowering systolic and diastolic blood pressure in comparison with various β-blockers.

One major advantage of α_1-blockers is that they are essentially free of significant adverse metabolic effects and can even reduce total cholesterol, low-density lipoprotein cholesterol and triglycerides and increase high-density lipoprotein cholesterol. Although the relevance of lipid changes to cardiovascular risk observed with these agents is not known, these changes are in sharp contrast to the adverse lipid effects of the thiazides and most β-blockers. Theoretically, the differences in lipid effects between antihypertensive drugs could have a major impact in determining the effectiveness of treatment regimens in the prevention of cardiovascular disease.

Prazosin, terazosin and doxazosin appear to have a similar likelihood of association with side-effects: in long-term trials about 10–15% of patients were withdrawn because of adverse experiences. Frank syncopal episodes are rare (<1%): the 'first-dose phenomenon' has been greatly reduced by giving a small initial dose at bedtime. When compared with placebo, some rather frequent side-effects of doxazosin therapy are: dizziness or vertigo (11% vs 5% with placebo), sonnolence (5% vs 1%) and fatigue/asthenia (12% vs 6%); many of these side-effects are mild to moderate. Impotence, a common adverse effect observed with other antihypertensive agents occurs infrequently with α_1-inhibitor. Some weight gain (usually 1–1.5 kg) has often been observed.

S_2-serotonin receptor antagonists

Ketanserin, the only available oral antagonist of S_2-HT (serotonin) receptors with some admixture of α_1-receptor blockade is a successfully used antihypertensive agent which causes blood pressure reduction by decreasing total peripheral resistance.

In spite of its recent introduction for the treatment of hypertension ketanserin has already been administered to vast numbers of patients with mild to moderate hypertension. It has been shown that ketanserin causes a blood pressure reduction greater than placebo and is equipotent to hydrochlorothiazide, β-blockers, calcium antagonists and ACE inhibitors. The most frequent side-effect is somnolence (7% vs 5% with placebo), while the incidence of dizziness, fatigue and gastrointestinal upset was similar to that found during placebo.

Ketanserin does not cause appreciable changes in glucose, lipoproteins and serum electrolytes and is not contraindicated in the presence of diabetes mellitus, congestive heart failure, peripheral vascular disease, chronic obstructive airway disease, gout and renal and hepatic failure.

SPECIFIC ASPECTS OF ANTIHYPERTENSIVE TREATMENT

Age

It has been suggested by some authors that age may influence the antihypertensive response to pharmacological treatment. Diuretics, calcium antagonists and ketanserin have been recommended for the treatment of elderly hypertensives; β-blockers and ACE inhibitors are claimed to do better in younger hypertensives, while α_1-inhibitors are neutral. There is not much to be gained by following these guidelines; efficacy is first and foremost related to pretreatment blood pressure levels.

General rules for all antihypertensive drugs prescribed to elderly hypertensives are: (see also Chapter 5).

RULES FOR TREATING THE OLDER HYPERTENSIVE

* Start with half the usual adult dose
* Titrate the dose on standing blood pressure
* Increase dosage after longer intervals

Race

Black hypertensives are less responsive to β-blockers and ACE inhibitors than white ones, while there are no convincing differences in the responses to diuretics, calcium antagonists, ketanserin and α_1-inhibitors. It has been presumed that the blood pressure elevation in black people is volume dependent and tends to coincide with rather low renin levels. This pattern is thought to be responsible for the greater responsiveness in blacks to some drugs than to others.

Physical exercise

While physical activity based on static exercise is contraindicated in all hypertensive patients because of the concomitant rise in total peripheral vascular resistance, physical activity based on dynamic exercise may be allowed at non-competitive levels. In hypertensive patients who like to exercise, calcium antagonists, ACE inhibitors and diuretics can be administered without special precautions while β-blockers should rather be avoided. The rationale is that the first group of antihypertensive agents does not interfere with the physiological rise in cardiac output and decrease in total peripheral resistance which characterises the haemodynamic response to dynamic exercise. By contrast, β-blockers can attenuate the physiological rise in systolic blood pressure in response to dynamic exercise by limiting the increase in output. This implies that the rise in muscle blood flow falls short of the requirements. Hence physical performance and endurance are likely to be interfered with.

Pregnancy

At the present time only α-methyldopa and β-blockers have been shown to reduce maternal and fetal events during pregnancy-induced hypertension. For further details see Chapter 5.

STRATEGY OF ANTIHYPERTENSIVE THERAPY

Once it has been demonstrated that the patient has sustained blood pressure elevation, the physician has to decide on treatment, starting with a non-pharmacological programme, but then proceeding to using drug treatment in order to normalize blood pressure as much as possible. This procedure aims at preventing, at least partially, hypertension-related cardio-vascular complications.

There is no doubt that the most rational approach would be to match the pharmacological properties of the drug under consideration with the pathophysiological profile of the individual patient. However, as it has already been argued, we are still far from establishing hypertensive mechanisms in a given patient. Arterial pressure is regulated through a complex of factors and even the assessment of only a few of these in the average hypertensive patient is hardly conceivable. A classification of hypertensives on the basis of a few arbitrary parameters is both premature and misleading.

The other side of the coin is equally unclear, in that there are still many uncertainties in identifying the mechanisms of action of antihypertensive drugs, and the more so because a number of them have multiple pharmacological properties.

The failure to correctly match the drug's properties to the patient's pathophysiological profile has given rise to the other extreme of applying a stepped-care approach. The basic concept behind step-care programmes is that what really matters in antihypertensive treatment is blood pressure reduction, not the means or mechanisms by which blood pressure is reduced. Therapy should be simple, starting generally with a single drug at low dose and only later if necessary progressing to more complex therapeutic regimens. Additional requirements are that the lowering of blood pressure should be gradual and that the drugs chosen are likely to be efficacious, with a minimum of discomfort.

As mentioned before, the first stepped-care programme proposed in 1977 by the US Joint National Committee on Detection and Treatment of High Blood Pressure (Fig. 1), offered a very limited choice at the first step (thiazides), with the suggestion that doses of thiazide should be increased quite substantially before resorting to an additional agent. Although justified on the basis of a favourable cost/benefit ratio when compared with the drugs available at that time, this stepped-care programme with only one drug at the first step was too rigid; only one year later (1978) the WHO Committee formulated more flexible recommendations (Fig. 2), suggesting a first step choice between a thiazide diuretic or a β-blocker.

Since 1978 additional experience has challenged some of these elementary notions of stepped care. As has been mentioned earlier in this chapter, the incidence of side-effects caused both by diuretics and β-blockers was worse than expected when the Medical Research Council Trial results were examined.

Furthermore, one has become aware that antihypertensive treatment by conventional drugs failed to reduce all types of cardiovascular events; in this respect some concerns have arisen about the unwanted metabolic effects of diuretics and to a minor extent of β-blockers.

Finally, during the last 10 years a great deal of information has become available with regard to the efficacy, security and tolerability of new classes of antihypertensive drugs, notably ACE inhibitors and calcium antagonists; such new findings have to be taken into account when guidelines for antihypertensive treatment are formulated.

These considerations recently resulted in a more liberal approach to the treatment of hypertension (Fig. 3.). The first step of treatment has now been amplified to include both calcium antagonists and ACE inhibitors, which facilitates the choice by the practitioner.

In view of these expanded options the question arises whether there are still some guidelines for the selection of the first drug. As mentioned, the first-step antihypertensive drugs are equipotent and therefore their efficacy per se cannot serve as a guideline. The choice among these various classes will therefore be made on the simple clinical evaluation of contraindications or indications in terms of comorbidity for the various compounds in the patient. The main points related to current antihypertensives have been summarized opposite.

When patients have uncomplicated mild to moderate hypertension without concomitant risk factors, the practitioner is obviously free to choose. He may tend to rely on the following considerations: 1) based on the results of controlled prognostic trials the choice will be a diuretic or a β-blocker, 2) if he is inclined to avoid adverse effects, his preference may go to ACE inhibitors, 3) if he is particularly concerned about the possible consequence of metabolic effects, the choice will vacillate between calcium antagonists, ACE inhibitors, α_1-inhibitors and ketanserin, 4) if he is preoccupied with the cost for the individual or society, a thiazide may rank first.

COEXISTING DISEASES OR HYPERTENSIVE COMPLICATIONS AS CRITERIA FOR INDIVIDUAL FIRST CHOICE OF ANTIHYPERTENSIVE THEERAPY

* *Diabetes mellitus*
  Avoid: Thiazides (and β-blockers?)
  Prefer: ACE inhibitors, calcium antagonists

* *Chronic obstructive bronchial disease*
  Avoid: β-Blockers
  Prefer: Calcium antagonists

* *Peripheral obstructive arterial disease*
  Avoid: β-Blockers (unless with ISA)
  Prefer: Calcium antagonists, S_2-antagonists

* *Ischaemic heart disease and ventricular ectopic beats*
  Avoid: Thiazide?
  Prefer: β-Blockers, calcium antagonists

* *Congestive heart failure*
  Avoid: β-Blockers
  Prefer: ACE inhibitors, calcium antagonists (dihydropyridines), diuretics

* *Impaired renal function*
  Avoid: β-Blockers, thiazides
  Prefer: Calcium antagonists, ACE inhibitors (small doses), loop diuretics

* *Left ventricular hypertrophy*
  Avoid: Vasodilators (hydralazine)
  Prefer: β-Blockers, calcium antagonists, ACE inhibitors

UP-STEPPING, SIDE-STEPPING, DOWN-STEPPING

When monotherapy with one of the first-step drugs, chosen according to the criteria above, does not normalize blood pressure, one can step-up to the second and eventually to the third step by adding one or two drugs (Fig. 4).

143

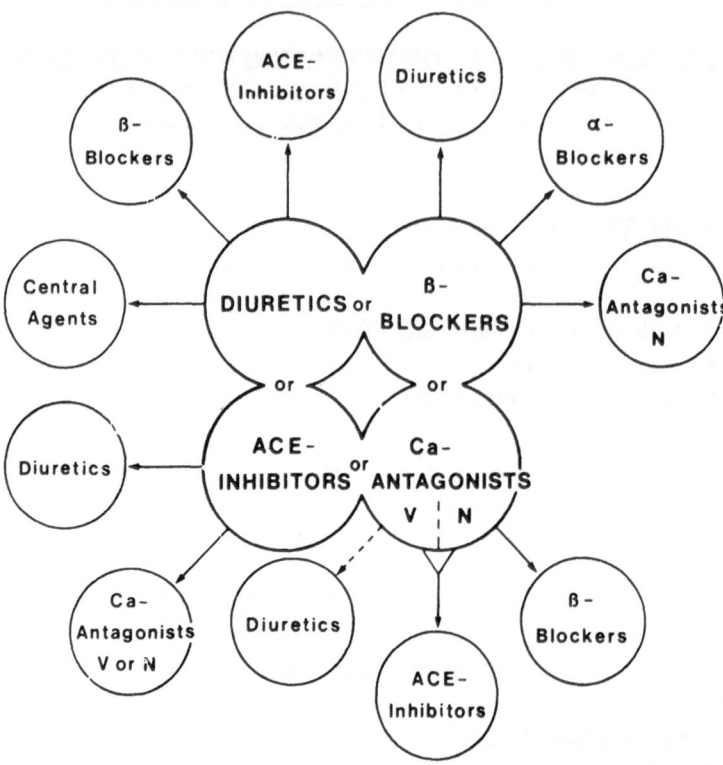

Fig. 3. Liberal stepped-care programme. Treatment is usually started with one of the four classes of agents indicated in the centre of the figure. The arrows indicate the possible additional drugs. (From Zanchetti A Step-wise treatment: which treatment first? In Strasser T, Ganten D (eds.) *Mild Hypertension: From Drug Trials to Practice.* Raven, New York, pp. 243–249

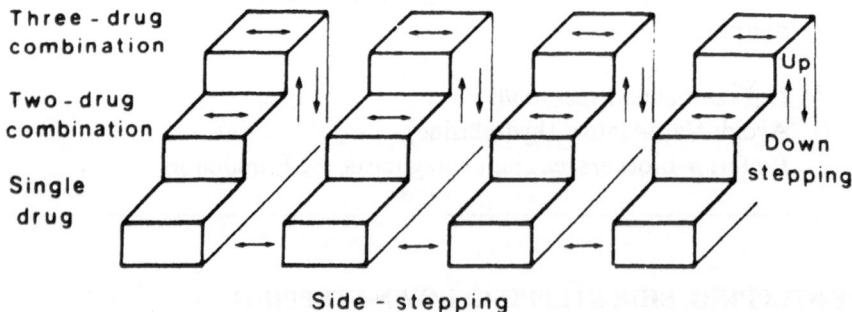

Fig. 4. Step-wise treatment of hypertension represented as an assay of parallel staircases with possibilities for up-stepping, side-stepping and down-stepping at each step (From Zanchetti A. (1990): Stepwise treatment in hypertension. In Ganten D and Mulrow PJ (eds.) *Pharmacology of Antihypertensive Therapeutics* Berlin/Heidelberg/New York: Springer-Verlag, pp. 741–763

The most important principles which are recommended for combinations are: 1) to combine drugs with different pharmacodynamic profiles, 2) to add a drug which can correct the counter-regulatory side-effects of the first one. In this way, we face no less than four staircases with a different antihypertensive agent as the first step and different combinations at the second and third steps.

Unlike the antiquated step-care approach (when it was only possible to move up) the present liberal approach allows for side-stepping and even down-stepping. Side-stepping, that is passing from one staircase to another, is advised when the blood pressure reduction during monotherapy or a subsequent combination appears to be less than satisfactory or when side-effects are unacceptable.

Down-stepping is called for when the reduction in blood pressure is beyond expectations or when adverse events are worse than expected.

This strategy has obvious advantages in terms of an individualized approach, while retaining some of the useful elements of protocolized medicine.

DURATION OF ANTIHYPERTENSIVE THERAPY

While down-stepping is a correct procedure under the circumstances indicated above, the question remains how often this may lead to ultimate cessation of therapy, assuming the blood pressure has stayed on a normal level for a long period. This issue is both of practical and theoretical interest for obvious reasons.

From the analysis of available studies, where antihypertensive therapy has been withdrawn after a long period of 'normalized' diastolic blood pressure (defined in different studies from <100 mmHg to ⩽85 mmHg), it appears that in almost all studies a proportion of previously treated patients maintain normal blood pressure values after treatment withdrawal. The proportion of 'cured' normalized patients is probably less than reported in most studies because the results critically depend on the duration of follow-up, which amounted to one year at the most in quite a number of studies.

The idea that adequate antihypertensive therapy in the long term might reverse the hypertension process has been negated by the evaluation of mild hypertension trials. The Australian Trial has shown that some 50% of patients randomized to the placebo group exhibited a spontaneous decline to normal pressure levels in the course of several years. The Medical Research Council reported a follow-up analysis showing that after withdrawal of active treatment and replacement by placebo, average blood pressure reached similar values to those in patients maintained continuously on placebo for 3–9 months.

It is therefore likely that most of the mild hypertensive patients who remain normotensive several months after withdrawal from active treatment are those who would have become normotensive anyway and therefore have been wrongly labelled as hypertensives in the first place.

Nevertheless, blood pressure may still remain normalized due to long-term treatment in a limited number of cases. There are plenty of theoretical mechanisms to account for this. The arterial baroreflex may have been reset to normal pressure levels. In addition, a regression of the structural components of hypertension, such as myocardial or vascular hypertrophy, may have occurred.

Selected references

Amery A, Birkenhäger W, Brixko P et al. (1985): Mortality and morbidity results from the European Working Party on High Blood Pressure in the Elderly trial. Lancet 1: 1349–1354.

Brunner HR, Nussberger J, Waeber B (1985): The present molecules of converting enzyme inhibitors. J Cardiovasc Pharmacol 7 (suppl 1): S2–S11.

Curb JD, Maxwell MH, Schneider KA et al. (1986): Adverse effects of antihypertensive medications in the Hypertension Detection and Follow-up Program. Prog Cardiovasc Dis 29 (suppl 1): 73–78.

Finnerty FA (1984): Step-down treatment of mild systemic hypertension. Am J Cardiol 53: 1304–1307.

Freis ED (1986): How diuretics lower blood pressure. Am Heart J 106: 185–187.

1988 Joint National Committee. The 1988 Report of the Joint National Committee on detection, evaluation and treatment of high blood pressure. Arch Int Med 148: 1023–1038.

Licht JH, Haley RJ, Pugh B, Lewis SB (1983): Diuretic regimens in essential hypertension. A comparison of hypokalemic effects, blood pressure control and cost. Arch Int Med 143: 1694–1699.

MacMahon SW, Cutler JA, Furberg OD, Payne CH (1986): The effects of drug treatment for hypertension on morbidity and mortality from cardiovascular disease. A review of randomized controlled trials. Prog Cardiovasc Dis 29 (suppl 1): 99–118.

MacMahon SW, Peto R, Cutler Y et al. (1990): Blood pressure, stroke and coronary heart disease. Lancet 1: 765–774.

Medical Research Council Working Party (1985): MRC trial of treatment of mild hypertension. Principal results. Br Med J 291: 97–104.

Medical Research Council Working Party (1988): Stroke and coronary heart disease in mild hypertension: risk factors and the values of treatment. Br Med J 296: 1565–1570.

Middeke M, Weisweiler P, Schwandt P, Holzgreve H (1987): Serum lipoproteins during antihypertensive therapy with β-blockers and diuretics: a controlled long-term comparative trial. Clin Cardiol 10: 94–98.

WHO/ISH (1983): Guidelines for the treatment of mild hypertension. Bull WHO 61: 53–56.

Zanchetti A (1987): Current drug treatment of hypertension: problems and perspectives. Ann Life Ins Med 81: 149–155.

Zanchetti A (1990): Stepwise treatment of hypertension. In: Ganten D, Mulrow PJ (eds.) Handbook of Experimental Pharmacology, Vol. 93, Pharmacology of Antihypertensive Therapeutics. Berlin: Springer-Verlag, pp. 741–763.

CHAPTER 9

Predictability, assessment and improvement of compliance with regard to taking antihypertensive drugs

GASTON E. BAUER

INTRODUCTION

The ultimate goal of antihypertensive treatment is the reduction and abolition of the excess mortality and morbidity associated with chronically elevated high blood pressure. Although the increased incidence of cardiovascular disease due to arterial hypertension has been known and appreciated since the introduction of blood pressure measuring devices, the benfits of blood pressure reduction have only been accepted during the past two decades, since the publication of major clinical trials involving ten thousands of hypertensive subjects.

The achievements have indeed been nothing short of impressive.

DIVIDENDS FROM ANTI-HYPERTENSIVE TREATMENT

* A marked fall in overall and especially cardiovascular mortality
* A striking decrease in cerebrovascular accidents
* Virtual abolition of hypertensive heart failure
* The virtual disappearance of malignant hypertension as a complication of primary hypertension
* Diminution in the risk of dissecting aneurysm
* Significant protection from progressive renal failure
* Reduction in diabetic vascular complications
* Arguably a delay in the development of ischaemic heart disease

---

Several important obstacles in the successful control of hypertension in the community remain to be overcome:

CURRENT PROBLEMS IN HYPERTENSION CONTROL

* Recognition and detection
* Referral for appropriate assessmemt
* Selection and initiation of suitable management
* Ensuring long-term adherence to therapy

The methods of detection, referral, initial assessment and introduction of therapy are important factors in facilitating, or mitigating against, long-term successful management.

COMPLIANCE

Definition and measurement of compliance

The term 'compliance' has been criticized by clinicians, epidemiologists and patients because of its authoritarian ambiance and the perception of compulsion. However, none of the alternatives, such as 'adherence to therapeutic regimens' or 'following treatment advice', have found wide acceptance in the medical and general community.

The definition of compliance has also been the subject of debate. Simple statements such as 'the extent to which a patient's health behaviour follows medical advice' or 'coincides with clinical prescription' seem explicit but place the entire responsibility on the consumer. A recent definition, 'compliance is the degree of co-operation between clinician and patient in the management of regimens, characterized by the patient's understanding of and adherence to these regimens including appropriate reporting back to the clinician', has been suggested to ensure that the physician shares in the success or failure of the patient's ability or willingness to follow treatment advice.

Measurement of adherence to treatment is also a difficult subject. Non-compliance either means that the patient has failed to keep follow-up appointments without explanation or that there is good reason to believe that he or she has not followed the prescribed treatment. Estimates of non-compliance vary greatly, from 20–80%, with the majority of reported studies falling in the 25–50% range. In a Boston teaching hospital outpatient

148

clinic, 50% of newly diagnosed and 30% of previously identified hypertensives failed to return within 6 months. In a Manhattan private practice, 51% of hypertensive subjects failed to reappear after their initial visit. In subsidized and strictly supervised trials, lower drop-out rates can be achieved. In the Australian National Blood Pressure Study, 3972 subjects were enrolled in the trial. Within 24 months, 1154 (29%) were withdrawn, of which 636 (16%) were patient initiated (Table 1).

Table 1. Withdrawals from treatment within 24 months (Australian National Blood Pressure Study)

Subjects screened	103 228	
Subjects enrolled in trial	3 972	
Withdrawals:		
Pressure limit exceeded (DBP > 110 mmHg)	174	4.3%
Intercurrent medical conditions	76	1.9%
Treatment transferred to family physician	268	6.8%
Patient-initiated withdrawal	636	16.0%
Total	1154	29.0%

Much more difficult than attendance is the measurement of how many subjects follow advice concerning life-style readjustments or take their prescribed medication with reasonable regularity. Progress has been made in the control of mutable risk factors, especially in the United States, Canada, Western European countries, Australia and New Zealand. Population surveys and trends in cardiovascular mortality statistics support this contention. However resistance from individual subjects and especially from financially interested industrial groups such as the tobacco industry remain to be overcome. 'Health before profits' is still a utopian concept in our free-trade society.

Adherence to pharmacological treatment is difficult to measure. In a well-defined group, such as the Canadian steel workers studied by the McMaster group, 50% of treated hypertensive subjects were estimated to have taken 80% or more of the prescribed drugs. Systematic or random pill counts are impracticable and unreliable as a measure of regular compliance with drug prescriptions. Blood levels, such as assays which can be used to monitor therapy with digoxin, are not available for any of the antihypertensive medications. Biochemical variations, including hypokalaemia or hyperuricaemia with the use of diuretics, are too insensitive and non-specific to be of clinical use. Blood pressure responses, which correlate with the taking of antihypertensive medication in large groups of subjects, lack sensitivity as well as specificity to be useful as short-term indicators of compliance.

Recently, patient self-reporting of regular or irregular intake of prescribed medication has again been advocated as a measure of compliance. Improvements in designing a suitable questionnaire or structuring the physician's enquiry during patient visits by presenting questions in a non-judgemental way, for example, "Some patients have had difficulty in taking these pills. Have you been able to take them on a regular basis?" may be helpful.

Factors influencing compliance

Plenty of factors mitigate against good compliance with drug treatment.

OBSTACLES TO COMPLIANCE

* Long duration of treatment
* A symptom-free disorder
* Absence of immediate or early subjective benefit
* The need for regular re-examinations
* Frequent and multiple drug administration
* Possible treatment side-effects
* Anxieties concerning long-term adverse metabolic effects
* Cost of treatment

Hypertension seems to be the very disorder which scores strongly on all or most of these adverse factors. Each and every point is predictive of poor adherence to continuing treatment. In infectious diseases a course of antibiotic administration may last for one or two weeks. In hypertension it will be years, if not life long.

Except in the malignant phase, or after the occurrence of vascular complications, hypertension is a symptom-free disorder. The majority of so-called hypertensive symptoms, such as headaches, epistaxis, and subtle behavioural or neuropsychiatric changes, are non-specific and randomly distributed over a wide range of blood pressure. The hypertensive patient cannot expect immediate or early subjective benefit, such as the rapid pain relief with appropriate treatment observed in patients suffering from acute gout. The only obvious short-term benefits of blood pressure reduction are apparent in the treatment of acute hypertensive crises, malignant hypertension and left ventricular failure, or in a different sense with job applications or licensing requirements which are barred to subjects with uncontrolled hypertension.

Hypertensive subjects, irrespective of their current treatment status, require regular supervision assessment and advice in order to reduce excessive cardiovascular mortality and morbidity. Visits to the physician's office may cause inconvenience and resistance which has to be overcome by patient explanation. The drug treatment of hypertension may become complicated with the need for two or more different pharmaceutical agents, administered several times per day. Medication to overcome drug-induced metabolic changes, such as potassium supplements, lipid-lowering agents, uricosuric agents, as well as treatment for associated disorders and the almost ubiquitous aspirin tablet, are frequently prescribed and expected to be taken on a regular basis. No wonder that compliance with treatment, which, at the time of the initial discovery of a mildly raised blood pressure, seemed a simple problem, rapidly becomes a nightmare. Side-effects attributed to a particular treatment regimen plus the concern about possible long-term metabolic disturbances are further circumstances which have been identified as interfering with compliance. Finally, long-term drug treatment significantly adds to the cost, whether it be borne by the individual or by the community.

Strategies to improve compliance

The achievement of a high level of compliance is very much part of the responsibility of the treating clinician. Further reductions in cardiovascular mortality can only be expected if the medical profession accepts the need to be fully involved in the prevention as well as treatment of common disorders. High blood pressure, high cholesterol and smoking are obvious examples. Physicians play the key role in the early detection and assessment as well as long-term supervision of hypertensive subjects. Physicians need to educate patients, prepare them for continuing treatment and monitor their progress at regular intervals.

> ## HOW TO IMPROVE COMPLIANCE
>
> * Patient education
> * Establishing close physician–patient rapport
> * Simplicity of treatment regimens
> * Attention to socioeconomic factors

Patient education

Patient education is the corner-stone of successful treatment and remains . primarily the responsibility of the supervising physician. An intelligent and complying patient will want to know the cause, the consequences and the likely outcome of his or her condition. Management of drug therapy requires the patient to have some knowledge of the pharmacological characteristics, the mode of action, possible side-effects and long-term metabolic consequences of the medication. In many communities the need for such information is part of the legal obligation placed upon the treating physician. The amount of detail conveyed to the patient may well depend on circumstances which are difficult to define but are obvious to the experienced clinician. The detail of educational material required for an individual subject may only become apparent after several interviews. There are few effective short cuts to adequate patient education. Pamphlets, brochures and books for use by patients are available from professional organizations. Some physicians prefer to prepare their own printed material.

Group sessions may be useful ancillary teaching aids, especially if combined with creating awareness of strategies for the control of other risk factors, including dietary advice, a stop-smoking campaign and exercise prescriptions. The experience of setting up a cardiovascular education centre has been an interesting one which can be recommended to become part of any institution involved in treatment and prevention of cardiovascular disease.

A specific aspect of hypertension education relates to the use of self-monitoring blood pressure devices. Whilst home blood pressure measurements are not mandatory for the management of subjects with mild to moderate hypertension, the technique can be very useful to patients who appear to be resistant to standard drug therapy. Frequently home blood pressure measurements record lower values than casual readings in the physicians office or the hospital hypertension clinic. The transient pressor effect of the physician, often perceived as a white-coated authoritarian figure, has been known for many years and confirmed by continuous blood pressure measurements. Portable automated cuff sphygmomanometers are available and in use in hypertension clinics and cardiovascular education centres (see also Chapter 1).

Physician–patient rapport

Successful compliance with long-term treatment is greatly enhanced if continuity of supervision can be attained. All patients, especially those with chronic disorders requiring long-term and possibly life-long treatment, choose to be under the care of a clinician or therapist personally known to them. Everyone prefers to be seen by Dr X or by Nurse Y, rather than by an ever-changing employee of an institution or a clinic no matter how great its research reputation might be.

Appointments at mutually suitable times will help to ensure patient attendance. The tact and friendliness of the doctor's secretary or the appointment clerk can have a great impact on compliance. The doctor's office and the hypertension clinic are here to serve the patien; compliance is in jeopardy if conversations and actions suggest a reversal of this relationship. Great delays in seeing patients requiring repeated attendances should be avoided as far as possible, although no patient expects his or her physician to be always on time. Unusual delays should be explained with appropriate apologies and, as far as possible, recurrences prevented.

During repeat visits less time can be spent on routine examination. Pathology and laboratory tests are time and resource consuming and should be kept to a minimum consistent with good medical practice. More emphasis should be given to enhance patient education and risk factor control. The experienced physician will never gloss over questions prepared by patients. If it transpires that the patient suspects that certain symptoms may be side-effects of prescribed treatment, sufficient time must be given to investigate and discuss the possibility. The wise practitioner will always be prepared to change medication if this can be done safely and without prejudice to good blood pressure control, even if fully aware that many patients find it more convenient to blame the treatment for certain complaints which appear to be anxiety or age related.

Appointment non-attenders should be tactfully contacted without being made to feel that they are not fully entitled to persevere or discontinue treatment. In this regard it is pertinent to be reminded that the most frequent cause of failure to comply is non-comprehension by the patient of information given, be it due to lack of time or inappropriate style.

Simplicity of treatment regimens

Adherence to prescribed treatment is enhanced by simple treatment regimens. Evidence is available that drug prescriptions which allow a once or at most twice daily administration are much more likely to be persevered with than medication requiring three or more doses per 24 hours. This has been confirmed for many chronic conditions including epilepsy and depressive states as well as cardiovascular disorders. In the treatment of hypertension, a drug which must be taken three or more times a day is unlikely to gain patient acceptability. The midday doses are the ones which are most commonly omitted. The trend for many pharmacological agents with short half-lives to be marketed in slow-release preparations has been helpful.

Many antihypertensive drugs are currently competing for acceptance as the drug of first choice, a topic discussed in Chapter 8. Experience from the major clinical trials suggest that no more than 50% of patients with mild and moderate hypertension can be adequately controlled with a single antihypertensive agent. Drug combinations have been established for many years and provide a very satisfactory form of treatment. Best known among these are the concurrent use of β-blockers and diuretics, angiotensin converting enzyme inhibitors and diuretics as well as combinations of a thiazide diuretic with a potassium-sparing compound. The use of combination preparations, however, limits the choice of the prescribing physician in terms of the balance of the individual compounds.

Mention has been made of the need to warn patients of side-effects which may cause concern unless anticipated. Headaches, flushing and oedema with some of the calcium-channel blockers, and cough with angiotensin converting enzyme inhibitors, are examples where a warning in time may ensure compliance with treatment and indeed enhance the patient's confidence in his treating physician.

Patients, now being much better informed about their medication than they were a decade or two ago, may express concern about the long-term safety of some antihypertensive agents because of their potential metabolic side-effects. It is the physician's duty to convey the most reliable information on the subject available to him. It seems unfortunate that non-compliance with and distrust of certain antihypertensive compounds may be the result of a campaign by a rival pharmaceutical firm in the course of promoting its own compound. How much better it would be if the original provider of the drug in question could be persuaded to inform the medical profession and, if necessary, the public, of any serious doubts which may have been cast on its produce, rather than wait for a tough competitor to do so. Safety in prescribing and indeed in pharmacology and therapeutics, depends on close co-operation between the pharmaceutical industry, the medical profession and the regulatory authorities. None can function to advantage without the others. This co-operation, within the framework of healthy competition, should also prevail within the pharmaceutical industry.

Socio-economic factors

The cost to consumer of drug treatment varies from country to country depending on a variety of circumstances including the degree of subsidization by the government authorities. In all free-economy societies, the medical profession has accepted the challenge of acting responsibly in terms of cost-effectiveness. Other factors being equal, the treating physician should select the least costly pharmaceutical agent suitable for the particular patient. This should be the rule whether the bulk of the cost is borne by the individual patient or by the community at large. The more expensive drug must have clearly identifiable advantages over the equally effective cheaper agents.

The cost of antihypertensive drug therapy will be least felt by the very poor and by the well-to-do. The indiginous underprivileged patients are likely to receive drugs free of charge or at a heavily subsidized and discount price, whilst, for the affluent, health expenditure tends to be a relatively small budget item.

The risk of not pursuing adherence to treatment

The detection of hypertensive subjects, be it by a physician or by community screening, has been widely discussed. Less attention has been given to the known hypertensive subject who has interrupted treatment for whatever reason.

That discontinuation of supervised treatment may have serious results has become apparent from various 'trials'. In 1982 California eliminated its Medicaid programme (coded as Medi-Cal) in an attempt to contain rising health care costs. Medi-Cal recipients were poor and medically needy but not eligible for federal assisted programmes such as those for the aged, 65 years or older, the blind and the disabled. Responsibility for providing health care for Medi-Cal recipients was transferred to the counties who received a grant equivalent to 70% of the funds the state would have spent on the programme. The impact of termination of Medi-Cal on 215 patients who had attended the UCLA Medical Ambulatory Care Center, was studied by assessing their health status, including blood pressure prior to discontinuation of subsidized health care and six months later. A comparison group who continued to receive free medical care from federal assisted programmes was also followed. Among hypertensive Medi-Cal-supported adults, blood pressure control deteriorated during the six months follow-up period. The percentage of patients with good control (diastolic blood pressure at or less than 90 mmHg) diminished from 75% to 34%, while those with poor control (diastolic blood pressure above 100 mmHg) rose from 3% to 31%. No such trends were observed in the comparison group. The mean increase in diastolic blood pressure in the subjects whose Medi-Cal benefits had been withdrawn was 10 mmHg which, according to Framingham data, is equivalent to an increase in relative risk of cardiovascular events of 40%.

Still more striking was the alarming increase in stroke mortality observed in North Karelia, Finland, following a decrease in the intensity of antihypertensive drug treatment in the late seventies, again in an attempt to reduce health care expenditures. Because of the very high prevalence of cardiovascular mortality and morbidity, an effective network of publicly funded health centres had been set up in North Karelia, staffed by community nurses and supervised by regional medical officers. The baseline survey in 1972 revealed that only 29% of female hypertensive subjects were on treatment and the percentage of effectively treated hypertensives was only 5%. Proportional stroke mortality was 19%. By 1977 an improvement in hypertension-related conditions was observed. The percentage of hyper-tensive females on medication had increased from 29% to 69%, those effectively controlled from 5% to 41%. Proportional stroke mortality had dropped from 19% to 10%. Between 1977 and 1982 subsidized medical health services were restricted resulting in the deterioration of hypertension control and in increased stroke mortality. In 1982 the number of hypertensive females on treatment had dropped from 69% to 59% and those effectively treated from 41% to 33%. There was a substantial increase in proportional stroke mortality from 10% to 15%. Similar, but less impressive, trends were observed in males.

Such well-documented unfavourable effects of the interruption or reduction in intensity of antihypertensive treatment clearly make it necessary to exercise great caution in advocating withdrawal of antihypertensive treatment. Whilst this may occasionally be possible, under close supervision, long-term success will be the exception rather than the rule.

PREDICTING ADHERENCE TO ANTIHYPERTENSIVE TREATMENT

Predicting adherence to antihypertensive treatment has received increasing attention during the past twenty years. More than 700 studies have been published examining variables which may be helpful in identifying factors which enhance or prevent successful long-term compliance with prescribed treatment. These can be broadly grouped as relating to the subject, the therapeutic intervention and the supervising treatment team.

The hypertensive subject

The main reasons mitigating against long-term good adherence to antihypertensive treatment prescriptions have been discussed. It is not surprising that attempts at identifying compliant and non-compliant subjects have been met with a good deal of scepticism. More than 20 years ago it had been stated that hospital staff were no better than 50% accurate in predicting patients who would comply. At about the same time it was noted that senior physicians were, if anything, less successful than junior colleagues in identifying potential defaulters from treatment. The problem was confounded by the fact that subjective estimates by treating physicians proved to be grossly inaccurate. No wonder that experts continue to repeat statements such as "every patient is a potential defaulter and compliance can never be assumed" or "clinicians cannot out-perform the toss of a coin in predicting which patient will comply".

Nonetheless a profile of the defaulting patient is emerging. In the Australian National Blood Pressure Study and in the more recent study of the 'aware' untreated hypertensive subject in Georgia, younger patients, under the age of 50 years, especially males active in the workforce and responsible for supporting their families were found to be prone to discontinuing supervised treatment. Subjects managed with advice concerning life-style readjustments were more likely to default than those prescribed antihypertensive drugs. Subjects who had no other perceived medical problem and had not suffered from a vascular complication were less likely to continue the long-term medical treatment. In general, subjects whose hypertension was discovered by a patient-initiated visit to a physician were adhering better to treatment prescriptions than those discovered at work or community screening examinations. Shortened assessment protocols and reduced intervals to initiation of drug treatment were positive factors in ensuring compliance with therapeutic advice.

Elderly patients, contrary to earlier views, are relatively good in adhering to treatment instructions. This may be related to the greater prevalence of comorbidity, fewer socioeconomic barriers to long-term treatment and perhaps most importantly to the realisation of the greater iminence of major vascular complications.

The therapeutic intervention

The therapeutic intervention recommended for the control of hypertension will depend on several circumstances, especially the degree of blood pressure elevation. For the management of mild hypertension (diastolic blood pressure between 90 and 104 mmHg) repeated blood pressure measurements over a period of three to six months are usually recommended, in accordance with experience that in nearly half of the subjects the diastolic blood pressure will remain below 95 mmHg and the introduction of drug treatment can be safely deferred. If there is no fall in blood pressure, non-pharmacological interventions are generally recommended. This advice, while scientifically sound, may encourage defaulting from supervised management and should therefore only be followed if compliance in terms of office or clinic follow-up attendance, does not appear to be in jeopardy. Sufficient data are available to demonstrate that withdrawal from supervised treatment is most likely to occur within the first six months of diagnosis and in subjects offered non-pharmacological rather than pharmacological treatment.

Non-pharmacological treatment must be offered as a positive alternative to drug medication rather than be seen as a device for prevarication and procrastination. Life-style changes, including diet modifications, decreasing salt intake, cessation of smoking, weight reduction, alcohol modification, increasing physical exercise and relaxation strategies are for many individuals more difficult to comply with than the ingestion of a few tablets. To some, non-pharmacological treatment seems to resemble a life of self-denial, asceticism and lack of fun and pleasure. Whilst progress has been made in the adoption of healthier life-styles with obvious benefit to cardiovascular fitness, a great deal of education is still needed (see Chapter 7).

Drug treatment should be initiated with a detailed and frank explanation of the pharmacological action and possible side-effects. The aim should be to obtain blood pressure control with the smallest number of tablets since simple treatment regimens are more likely to be complied with. Changes in dosage and medication should be kept to a minimum and treatment with drugs, which to recent graduates may appear 'old fashioned', not altered if blood pressure control is satisfactory and side-effects not troublesome (see Chapter 8).

The evaluation and management of side-effects is one of the difficult aspects of antihypertensive drug treatment. Experience from large-scale placebo-controlled clinical trials has taught us that the complaint rate for such symptoms as fatigue, giddiness and lack of energy tends to be not significantly different in subjects on placebo and active hypertensive medication. Certainly, in the Australian National Blood Pressure Study, the withdrawal rate because of drug side-effects was similar in the active and control groups. The default in attendance rate over a two-year period was also similar in the two treatment groups and in the third group who were observed but did not receive tablets.

Patients with severe hypertension may have to be persuaded more strongly to accept side-effects of medication if alternative drugs prove ineffective in controlling blood pressure. In such instances, the educational message must be clearly delivered: the prime task is reduction in blood pressure; the secondary consideration is minimizing side-effects. The patient's intelligence and the physician's therapeutic skills are usually successful in overcoming such difficult clinical problems. Certainly no patient should be promised normalization of blood pressure without side-effects.

The 'therapeutic team'

The physician plays the major part in facilitating the patient's adherence to therapeutic advice. To do so, he or she will have to demonstrate to the patient that the overriding interest of the therapeutic team is to ensure success in controlling blood pressure and prevention of complications with the minimum interference with the patient's daily routine. Advice regarding life-style modifications and treatment prescription must be seen to be offered with due regard to the patient's expectations. The physician not only has to be up-to-date with the new advances in therapy but, equally important appear to be a caring and compassionate individual prepared to discuss problems perceived by the patient. The commodity most appreciated by patients and yet difficult to obtain, is time and attention. Once rapport is established the physician–patient relationship will be more easily maintained.

A nurse practitioner or a clinical pharmacist may be well equipped to take over the role of representing the therapeutic team, once the initial assessment has been carried out and treatment strategies devised. Again there is need to ensure continuity of patient contact with the additional provision of medical consultative services as required. Certainly such methods of health care delivery work very well in communities which, by the process of time and education, have accepted the system. The key to successful management of hypertensive patients by paramedical personnel is that it is perceived to be a stabilized norm rather than a cheaper substitute.

The pharmaceutical industry

The pharmaceutical industry plays a key role in the management of hypertension and has a vested interest in promoting compliance. The great advances in the pharmaceutical treatment during the past 40 years have been pioneered or perfected by the industry. An enormous investment in time, energy and money has resulted in a great choice of effective and acceptable antihypertensive medication. The industry, in addition to introducing new compounds through research developments, has played a major role in the dissemination of knowledge and other educational exercises.

The methods of commercial promotion have a significant impact on adherence to therapeutic advice. Positive advertising, emphasizing the advantages of the preparation under consideration, is a very useful and legitimate way of promotion providing that all claims are based on good scientific evidence and readily capable of substantiation. The responsibility to disseminate knowledge about adverse drug effects should be shared by the parent drug company, the regulatory authorities and the medical profession. Perhaps this may seem counsel of perfection but without such trust and self-criticism it seems difficult to expect improvements in patient's compliance with treatment advice.

PREDICTABILITY, ASSESSMENT AND RECOMMENDATIONS FOR IMPROVING ADHERENCE TO THERAPEUTIC REGIMENS

Predictability of adherence to treatment in a chronic and symptom-free disorder, such as hypertension, is difficult and must be recognized as of limited accuracy. Recent studies suggest that it may be better than 'the toss of a coin' but clearly more research is required. Gradually, factors which identify patients who are more likely to continue with treatment are being identified such as mature age and favourable socioeconomic conditions including family support. Special efforts can then be made to provide health education for subjects who are at greatest risk of defaulting.

The assessment of compliance presents a special problem. Subjective judgments by clinicians seem to have low reliability and 'experience' provides no guarantee of a superior result. Objective measurements are in their infancy, pill counts unreliable, blood and urine tests not available for routine use. Strategies of improving self-reporting may be worth while pursuing, but at all times can only be of limited value.

Improvement in adherence to treatment advice is one of the challenges in the community control of hypertension. No longer are we prepared to accept the '50% rule' which states that 50% of hypertensive subjects are aware of their condition; of these, 50% are on treatment; and, of these 50% are adequately controlled. In many communities hypertension control is now much better than 12.5%. The key to improvement must lie in education: education of the patient and his family as to the risks of uncontrolled

160

hypertension, the benefits and relative ease of treatment and the choices which are currently available; education of the physician and the therapeutic team, not only of the strategies of non-pharmacological interventions and the latest drugs available, but also the need to encourage and facilitate ongoing treatment (in spite of the fact that it may be labour-intensive, time-consuming and expensive); education of other interested parties, including the pharmaceutical industry, the government and other health regulatory bodies. The introduction of new agents must stress their positive advantages and place them in proper perspective in comparison with other drugs available. Steps should be taken to remove or reduce unreasonable penalties associated with the hypertension label in respect to employability, insurability and licensing requirements, such as driving public vehicles or flying aircraft.

The final reminder to the physician interested in looking after contented and complying hypertensive patients may well be: Treatment must be EFFECTIVE, SAFE, SIMPLE AND CHEAP.

Selected references

Blackwell B (1973): Drug therapy: patient compliance. *N Engl J Med* 287: 249.

Caron HS, Roth JP (1968): Patients' co-operation with a medical regime. *J Am Med Assoc* 203: 922–926.

Davis MS (1966): Variations in patient's compliance with doctors' orders. *J Med Educ* 41: 1037–1048.

Engelland AL, Alderman HH, Powell HB (1979): Blood pressure control in private practice: a case report. *Am J Public Health* 69: 25–29.

German PS (1988): Compliance and chronic disease. *Hypertension* II (Suppl II): II56–II60.

Gillum RF, Neutra RR, Stason WB *et al.* (1979): Determinants of dropout rate among hypertensive patients in an urban clinic. *J Community Health* 5: 94–100.

Haynes RB, Taylor DW, Sackett DL (Eds.) (1979): *Compliance in Health Care.* Johns Hopkins University Press, Baltimore.

Lurie N, Ward NB, Shapiro MF *et al.* (1984): Termination from Medi-Cal – does it affect health? *N Engl J Med* 311: 480–484.

McClellan WM, Hall WD, Brogan D *et al.* (1988): Continuity of care in hypertension, an important correlate of blood pressure control among aware hypertensives. *Arch Int Med* 148: 525–528.

Management Comittee (1980): The Australian therapeutic trial in mild hypertension. *Lancet* 1: 1261–1267.

Morisky DE, Green LW, Levine DM (1986): Concurrent and predicitve validities of a self-reported measure of medication adherence. *Med Care* 24: 67–74.

Sackett DL, Haynes RB, Gibson ES *et al.* (1975): Randomised clinical trial of strategies for improving medication compliance in primary hypertension. *Lancet* 1: 1205–1207.

Tuomilehto J, Nissinen A, Puska P *et al.* (1985): Alarming increase in stroke mortality in middle-aged women associated with the decrease of antihypertensive drug treatment in the community. Abstract, Second European Meeting on Hypertension, June 1985.

Vetter H, Ramsey LE, Luscher TF, Schrey A, Vetter W (Eds.) (1985): Symposium on compliance – improving strategies in hypertension. Vol. 3 Suppl. 1.

Index